DIABETES *reach for health and freedom*

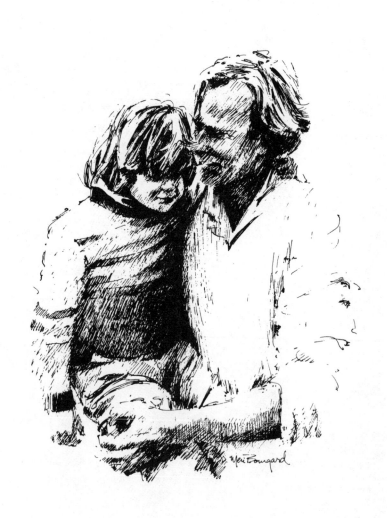

THE AMERICAN DIABETES ASSOCIATION

DIABETES *reach for health and freedom*

EDITED BY

DOROTHEA F. SIMS

American Diabetes Association National Board Member;
Co-Chairman, Committee on Health Care Delivery, National
Diabetes Advisory Board

prepared under the auspices of the Vermont Affiliate,
American Diabetes Association 1983–1984

CONTRIBUTORS

Margaret Calahan, R.D.
Madeleine Carleton, R.D.
Shelly Eurich, R.D.
Mary Ellen Henry, R.N.
Edward S. Horton, M.D.

Janet Moreland, R.N.
David C. Robbins, M.D.
Ethan A.H. Sims, M.D.
George W. Welsh III, M.D.
Debra Vinci, M.S., R.D.

Illustrations by Meri Bourgard

THE C.V. MOSBY COMPANY
ST. LOUIS • TORONTO   1984

Publisher: Thomas A. Manning
Editor: Nancy L. Mullins
Supervising editor: Karen A. Edwards
Manuscript editor: Margaret A. Weeter
Book design: Nancy Steinmeyer
Cover design: Diane M. Beasley
Production: Barbara Merritt, Linda R. Stalnaker

This is a revised edition of a
book previously published by
The C.V. Mosby Company under the
same title.

Printed in the United States of America

The C.V. Mosby Company
11830 Westline Industrial Drive, St. Louis, Missouri 63146

Library of Congress Cataloging in Publication Data

Main entry under title:

Diabetes: reach for health and freedom.

  At head of title: The American Diabetes
Association.
  "Prepared under the auspices of the Vermont Affiliate,
American Diabetes Association, 1983-1984."
  Includes bibliographical references and index.
  1. Diabetes. I. Sims, Dorothea F., 1916-
II. Calahan, Margaret. III. American Diabetes Associa-
tion. Vermont Affiliate.
RC660.D547 1984   616.4′62   83-23827
ISBN 0-8016-0163-0

F/VH/VH   9 8 7 6 5 4 3 2 1   03/B/332

FOREWORD

Dorothea Sims and a team of health professional associates have devised a consumer book about diabetes not only for the person with diabetes but for all health professionals who advise diabetic people. Anyone interested in diabetes should read it, but as Mrs. Sims says, "not all at one time." One might wonder whether another book on diabetes is needed. However, this book is unique, for its humanity adds a dimension to the usual education benefits and because a consumer has integrated the expertise of the professionals without diluting their science.

As a consumer, Mrs. Sims' positive attitudes are portrayed throughout the text. The perceptive reader will quickly see that this book is for the living and for the lively. The pedantics of the usual consumer book are transformed by infusing the experiences, wisdoms, and individualities of people with diabetes. The author insists that the person with diabetes first be considered a human being. Yet this humanism is nicely balanced by up-to-date information about the science of diabetes. Thus the text is a brilliant meld of high-quality science and sensitive art, a mix that must be achieved when helping the person with diabetes.

All who read *Diabetes: Reach for Health and Freedom* should try to emulate its philosophy and learn its science. The message is clear to those with diabetes: Continue to be the unique human being you are. Learn to cope wisely with diabetes so that you can grapple successfully with the more important challenges in life. Learn, strive, succeed, prevail. These are the verbs that should reflect your attitude toward diabetes.

The message to the health professionals is also clear. In addition to learning about modern methods of treatment, learn to appreciate your diabetic patients as people. Help them help themselves. Be ready to be of service but avoid being patronizing. Be appropriately positive and reluctantly negative.

The reader should enjoy the illustrations and their pithy comments; these serve as guideposts for the text. Note the repetitive emphasis on regular physical activity and the key importance of emotions. Since Mrs.

Sims is an articulate, humanistic person, both are discussed with great sophistication.

I hope each reader will enjoy this book and become imbued with its spirit. Life is for living. One cares for diabetes to live; one doesn't live to care for diabetes. We are shown how a person with diabetes not only survives but prevails. This book suggests how anyone can successfully cope with diabetes. The author would have everyone with diabetes do so.

Fred W. Whitehouse, M.D.

Chief, Division of Metabolic Disease, Henry Ford Hospital, Detroit, Michigan;
President, American Diabetes Association, 1978–1979

INTRODUCTION

The American Diabetes Association is proud to present this updated edition of *Diabetes: Reach for Health and Freedom*. The American Diabetes Association offers hope for tomorrow through research and help for today through education. This warm, sensitive book is a prime example of the best kind of help. The author has developed an informative and accessible guide that will be of practical value to persons with either insulin-dependent or non-insulin-dependent diabetes. The book also offers hope for tomorrow through its wise and human approach to the difficult problems of diabetes. Hope for persons with diabetes lies not only in potential breakthroughs in diabetes research but also in the small and large victories won daily by people who have consciously chosen to gain control of their lives and of diabetes. For these persons *Diabetes: Reach for Health and Freedom* will prove to be an invaluable resource and a good friend.

Allan L. Drash
President, American Diabetes Association,
1983-1984

PREFACE

A message to the people who help those who have diabetes and to the people who have to live with diabetes

The American Diabetes Association and its Vermont Affiliate offer you this book about the daily management of both insulin-dependent (Type I) and non-insulin-dependent (Type II) diabetes. We believe that the book is unique in five ways.

1. It is offered to both patients and professionals together. The "you" in the text refers to the person with diabetes. But the "we" refers to us all, authors, diabetics, and health professionals. We are all searching together for ways to manage the challenge of diabetes, and we have much to gain from sharing our knowledge and experience. So we hope we have written in a style and language that is clear and interesting to everyone. A common language helps a lot in learning new tasks. Of course, no one language will serve everyone's needs, and there is no use in reading alone, especially about such a difficult subject as diabetes. We hope that health professionals and diabetics will read this book together.

We believe that the diabetic should be able to look beyond survival to a productive and satisfying life, to work and play, to be a parent, and to make a contribution to our communities. Ideally the person with diabetes should have a physician who oversees and coordinates care and a nurse and diet counselor to help with the daily routines at home. Of course, in real life, the members of this team may vary according to where people live. But the person with diabetes is always the central figure, an equal partner in the team, actively developing a personally creative life with diabetes.

2. We hope that this book will alert health care people, people with diabetes, and their families to the preventive aspects of living successfully with diabetes. It is well known that both types of diabetes run in families. In the natural course of events, therefore, much can be done by both health professionals and persons with diabetes themselves to be on the lookout for diabetes in others. They can help to prevent it by sharing their knowledge and teaching good habits of nutrition and physical activ-

ity to close relatives. The relationships between diabetes and obesity and diabetes and heart disease are being studied very carefully. The more this knowledge can be shared, the fewer people there will be who develop diabetes.

3. It is now clearly recognized that there are two main types of diabetes and that their causes and treatments differ greatly. We emphasize this by separating the goals and daily routines for persons with non-insulin-dependent diabetes from those for insulin-dependent diabetics. In this way, each person learns just what applies to his or her particular type and stage of diabetes.

4. Wherever possible, we have given specific instructions in positive terms rather than a long list of "don'ts."

5. We have included more than the usual amount of information about how the body works in order to help us all appreciate it and have realistic goals about it. We believe that people who have diabetes both need and want to understand the reasons behind the necessary changes in their lives.

We hope that this book provides materials that can serve as background for making choices in treatment. All the methods and routines described here are in varying use by different people in different centers throughout the United States. However, this book is not intended to be a substitute for guidance by the physician. In fact, persons with diabetes should always ask to go over any educational materials about diabetes with the health professional most closely involved with their care. In this way they can make the best use of the information in their individual situations.

Like many good ideas, the need for this book was identified in two different places at the same time. In the summer of 1975, members of the nursing and dietary staff of the Medical Center Hospital of Vermont formed a committee to write an educational packet to help people with diabetes when they returned home and to ensure that there would be a standard reference for use throughout the hospital.

In the meantime, I had been working as a Fellow in Health Care at the Radcliffe Institute to develop a new educational approach to meet the lifelong needs of people with diabetes. My aims were to share an up-to-date understanding of how the body handles fuels to provide energy and to teach techniques of decision making by offering practical choices in treatment plans.

The physicians of the Metabolic Unit of the College of Medicine at the University of Vermont worked long and hard on this project and supported the concept of an interdisciplinary group effort that would include "consumer" skills. I have had insulin-dependent diabetes for 25 years and know many other people with diabetes.

From November 1975 to January 1977, under the auspices of the Vermont Affiliate of the American Diabetes Association, the following persons worked on this project with me:

Margaret Calahan, R.D.	Edward S. Horton, M.D.
Madeleine Carleton, R.D.	Janet Moreland, R.N.
Shelly Eurich, R.D.	Ethan A.H. Sims, M.D.
Mary Ellen Henry, R.N.	George W. Welsh III, M.D.

At that time, a short version in a loose-leaf notebook was produced locally for Vermonters who have diabetes. By 1979, this notebook had been distributed widely throughout the country. It was then decided to revise and expand it for general publication. The result has been a valuable experience of mutual learning, bringing together the viewpoints and skills of nurses, dietitians, people with diabetes, and physicians who engage in both research and the care of patients. These people all made essential contributions, which I coordinated in my capacity as editor and writer and from my perspective as a diabetic.

Meri Bourgard's drawings express emotions common to all human beings. We all experience disbelief, anger, confusion, frustration, and fear. With the right support and education, we learn to balance these emotions with determination, curiosity, courage, and a creative acceptance resulting in independence. Diabetes intensifies the human struggle, and we are grateful for the perspective her drawings offer.

This edition of *Diabetes: Reach for Health and Freedom* is essentially a new book, a pleasant sign of the great progress made in knowledge, technology, and attitudes toward diabetes in the last four years. It is also a pleasure to welcome to the group of contributors two outstanding new authors, Debra Vinci, M.S., R.D., and David C. Robbins, M.D.

The entire effort would never have seen the light of day without the steady encouragement and technical assistance of Nancy Moreland and Nancy Perrine. The support of Joseph Mailloux of the hospital administration and the skilled work of Dick Armstrong in the Hospital Print Shop were essential to the production of our first 1000 copies. Many others helped along the way, especially the group of more than 30 pretest readers, many of whom were diabetic or had diabetes in their families.

This edition is dedicated to all the people who have helped me live with diabetes, but most especially to my husband Ethan, researcher, teacher, physician, and my personal guide, philosopher, and friend.

Dorothea F. Sims

CONTENTS

What can you expect from this book?

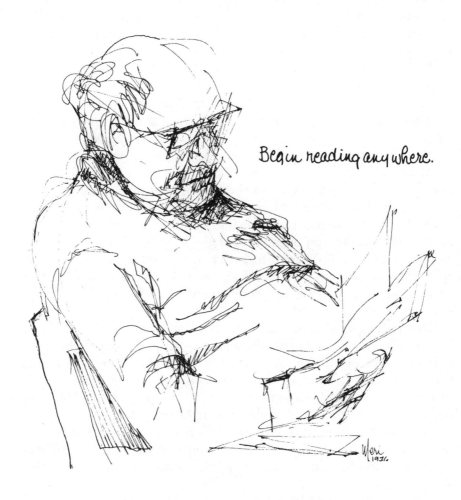

Begin reading any where.

Ask your doctor or nurse to go over this book with you because it will not tell *you* exactly what or when to eat or how much, if any, insulin you may need. Its aim is to share with you today's best understanding of what is happening in your body and to show you the principles behind the new tasks that living with diabetes calls for. It also will show you a whole range of choices about how you handle your diabetes on a daily basis.

In addition, you need the help of your *doctor, nurse,* and *diet counselor* to work out details of your daily plan, to be sure that you agree with your doctor about the information in this book, and to use it to help you live successfully with diabetes. Be sure that you know exactly what your doctor expects of you—and what you can expect of your doctor. The name of the game today is collaboration.

Remember that this book is only a small part of what will be available to you. It should be regarded as a friendly reference, not a rule book. No one can be expected to learn all about something as complex as the human body in a short time. Don't even try to read all of this book at once. But keep on trying to learn more, because *the more you know, the freer you will be of limitation.* You will find useful references in Appendix A.

More and more is being learned about diabetes. With modern technology we can begin to see in detail the systems in our bodies that relay information about our energy needs and release the energy available in food. We also know that human beings in many parts of the world can adapt and be healthy on different diets and in varied situations. For example, life in India is different from that in the United States, yet there are healthy people in both places. So it will not surprise you to find that there is more than one way for people to take care of themselves, with or without diabetes.

Each person with diabetes is different, not only in the sense that every human being is unique, but also because diabetes presents itself differently in each individual. Not only that, but as life goes along, our bodies naturally change and the diabetes changes too. Therefore, some of this material may be useful but some may not—at this point in your life. But you can start the good habit of learning right now.

You may have suggestions to make this book more useful with additions from your own experience. The person with well-controlled diabetes has a lot to offer. Share your knowledge! Above all, *never be afraid to ask questions.*

If you do not know a health professional who can help you, call your county medical society and ask for specialists in endocrinology, diabetes, or internal medicine. The Yellow Pages of the telephone book also lists

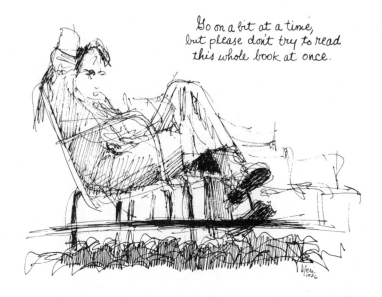

Go on a bit at a time,
but please don't try to read
this whole book at once.

specialists, and the local affiliate of the American Diabetes Association may be able to direct you to physicians most competent in the field of treating diabetes. Health resources vary somewhat from state to state, both in terms of what is available and how the resources are listed in telephone books. For example, when there is a national organization, such as the American Diabetes Association, it will probably be listed under American, with a local affiliate number as a subheading. In some states there is a section in front of the telephone book called *Guide to Services* that lists many voluntary health services. State departments of health are often good sources of information. In addition, hospitals are an excellent source of service and information about outpatient services. There is usually a section in the Yellow Pages listing regional hospitals.

Most states have home health agencies and visiting nurse associations as well as public health nursing offices, which are located throughout the regions.

State universities and colleges often have extension services with excellent nutritional resources as an important part of what they have to offer. Extension services are usually available by county.

Part 1
General considerations

Chapter 1
Understanding diabetes

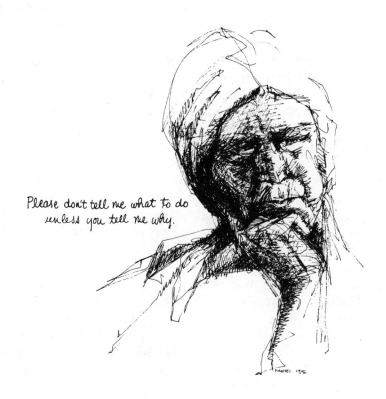

Please don't tell me what to do
unless you tell me why.

*Diabetes: 3000 B.C. to the
present revolution in
self-care*

The disease

Diabetes is one of the oldest known diseases. It was described and treated, though not very well, in Greece and India thousands of years ago. It is, at least in part, hereditary. But the human race has survived it and so can you.

The person who has diabetes has to think for the pancreas, one of the most complex organs in the body. Its job is to act as a traffic cop, working with the brain to direct the energy we get from our food to keep us at the right temperature, able to grow and heal and throw off infection, to love and work and respond to challenge, no matter if we are resting or running, hot or cold, well or ill, old or young. It is a miracle when you come to think of it. Not much wonder that we haven't found a cure and that, no matter how hard everyone tries, we are often confronted with failure. One of the chief goals of this book is to ease the burdens of guilt and fear so often associated with diabetes.

In diabetes, the body loses its normal ability to make use of the foods that are eaten, because the pancreas fails to produce enough insulin. The pancreas, a gland located just behind the stomach, produces hormones that regulate the use of the body's fuels. Two of these hormones, insulin from the beta cells and glucagon from the alpha cells, interact with each other to keep the level of available energy in the bloodstream just right.

Over centuries of evolution, the body has developed a system of checks and balances to keep us healthy. We eat a variety of foods to provide us with energy. Some foods are digested quite rapidly to give us immediate energy so we can act quickly at work, in sports, or in emergencies. These foods are the many kinds of starches and sugars, all of which are carbohydrates. Proteins and fats provide energy over longer periods for growth and healing and for the body to draw on when food is not available. Some of the energy in food (calories) is stored in the liver and muscles as glycogen and some is stored as body fat. We need some of all the different kinds of food to live a full and healthy life.

Each cell in the body can be compared to a tiny engine that uses a mixture of fuels, including glucose, fats, and proteins. Glucose is a simple sugar, the form to which complex starches and sugars are converted to circulate in the blood. Insulin is necessary to allow glucose (fuel) to enter most of the body's cells (engine) and be burned for energy. Glucagon acts to release the glucose from the glycogen stored in the liver when we have used up the glucose available in the blood.

Normally, insulin is delivered by the pancreas into the bloodstream at the time of eating so that the cells can absorb and burn or store the proper amount of fuel for whatever activity the body will be engaged in next. The pancreas also provides a small but steady supply of background insulin at all times. When the body manufactures too little insulin, glucose cannot be used or stored effectively. The potential energy in our food remains locked up. The body literally starves, and the unused glucose builds up in the blood and runs off in the urine. These two factors bring on the symptoms of diabetes.

Diabetes has two main types: Type I, insulin-dependent diabetes, and Type II, non-insulin-dependent diabetes. Type II is the most common in the United States today. Perhaps 80% of the more than 10 million Americans with diabetes have non-insulin-dependent diabetes, and most of them are adults who have gained extra weight. In Type II diabetes, the pancreas still produces insulin, as much or more than normal, but not enough to handle the food in a healthy way in the face of excess fat. Type II diabetes is in some ways less well understood in regard to causes and treatment than Type I. Perhaps people with Type II diabetes have inherited a tendency to store extra calories as fat and to develop a resistance to the action of their own insulin. It is clear that getting fat is not the single cause of diabetes, though it may combine with other factors to bring diabetes into the open. Research tells us that this kind of diabetes can often be dealt with by weight loss, increasing physical activity, and really limiting the amount of food eaten. But that means changing habits and lifestyles, a difficult feat in a country such as the United States where food is both abundant and available with little or no actual physical work. People with these inherited tendencies are at the mercy of our affluent, overfed, and sedentary culture. Type II diabetes is on the increase world-wide in industrialized societies.

Type I diabetes usually occurs in young, lean people. The pancreas has lost its ability to produce insulin, which must be replaced so that the body does not starve. That is why Type I is called insulin-dependent. Unfortunately, we do not yet have the technical capability of delivering insulin the way the body does naturally. The best ways we have today are injections of insulin 2 to 4 times a day or open-loop insulin pumps (see Chapter 12). Therefore the insulin-dependent diabetic must learn special skills, a sort of internal computer on duty 24 hours a day, to balance food intake, insulin injections, and energy output in all its forms, from resting to working and exercise. These skills are different from those needed to manage Type II diabetes. Therefore some of the chapters in this book are specially for Type I and others are just for Type II.

The revolution of the 1980s

Diabetes self-care in the 1980s is undergoing a revolution. We are in a time of hope, and it is now a realistic goal to "reach for health and freedom." Let's look at the history of diabetes treatments and the highlights of progress in the areas of research, technology, and attitudes during the last few years.

For nearly 5000 years, all that was known was that people with diabetes lost the sugar they ate into their urine. In the early 1900s, we learned that failure of the pancreas was the source of the disease. In 1910, Dr. Allen of New York devised "starvation diets" that eliminated sugars and starches completely from the diet. This treatment worked well for the overweight Type II diabetic whose pancreas was still producing insulin. But the diabetic whose pancreas did not produce any insulin did not survive for long. In 1921, insulin became available, saving the lives of thousands of Type I diabetics. For the last 50 years, both strict diets and insulin treatment have often been used for both types of diabetes. In fact, it is only recently that we have come to understand that the overweight diabetic usually does not need insulin and that the insulin-dependent diabetic does not need a sharply restricted diet.

In consequence, many people with diabetes have often been burdened by rigid rules that might not apply to their particular type and stage of diabetes. In addition, the person with diabetes usually was not encouraged to take responsibility for improving or modifying the treatment plan. There was a very good reason for this approach. There was no reliable way of keeping track of what was happening to blood glucose levels on an hour-to-hour basis. All we had to work with was urine testing, which is only an indirect and often inaccurate measure of blood glucose (see Chapter 4).

Now there are simple, accurate, and affordable techniques by which people with diabetes can monitor their own blood glucose wherever and whenever it is desirable, at home, at work, at school, or on vacation (see Chapter 4). For the first time, the person who lives with diabetes has the information everyone has been looking for: what happens to the blood in response to food, exercise, events and stresses of daily life, and insulin or oral agents, if needed.

This new technology became available just at the right time. Today, most people with diabetes are living lives of average length and they want to be active and healthy. Evidence is accumulating from research that strongly suggests that it is important for long-term health to keep the blood glucose as near normal as possible. We still don't have all the answers, but it is clear that prolonged high levels of blood glucose are harmful to the blood vessels and nerves that reach all parts of the body. There is a high rate of kidney failure, blindness, sexual problems, nerve damage, and certain types of vascular disease that are known to be associated with diabetes. These are called the long-term complications of diabetes (see Chapter 6). Fortunately, new treatment methods can minimize these complications. But, of course, it is best to avoid them in the first place. The most exciting areas of research show that normalizing blood glucose can sometimes prevent, postpone, or even reverse the damage to blood vessels and nerves. It is not yet known to what degree the blood glucose must be brought toward normal to avoid the complications. But most doctors today agree that it is worthwhile for everyone involved to work at managing diabetes as carefully as possible. Self–blood glucose monitoring (SBGM) is the key to success. See Chapter 4 for a detailed description of what's involved.

How you can be part of the revolution: "help for today"

The goal of treatment in diabetes is to keep the blood glucose within a range of 60 to 180 mg/dl as much of the time as possible for two reasons. First, people with diabetes feel better and enjoy life more when the diabetes is under control. Second, the nearly normal range avoids wide swings in blood glucose levels, which are both inconvenient and hazardous. But we have to face the fact that we do not yet have the perfect method of treating or "curing" diabetes, so the daily chores of living with diabetes don't always work. It is important to recognize that often, when things go wrong, it's not a question of "cheating" or poor health care—it's inadequate methods of care. Life is hard enough without feeling guilty when it's not appropriate, and most of us know well enough when it is appropriate. However, these very inadequacies mean that it is most important for your long-term health that you be informed about how your body works, up-to-date about the latest techniques for self-care, and able to be an equal partner on your health care team.

SBGM is having some unexpectedly beneficial effects on the relationships between physicians and persons who have diabetes. The doctor's prescription is being replaced by the idea that the doctor shares decision making with the person who has diabetes. Those who are testing their blood glucose are saying, "Things make sense for the first time. Now I can see what works and why." That sense of personal responsibility and understanding is opening the door to negotiating a treatment plan that is based on shared up-to-date information unique to each individual. The daily plan can take into account not only the type and stage of diabetes but also the characteristics and personal preferences of each person. When people share in making decisions about their daily lives, they are much more likely to want to stick to those decisions. Many doctors and nurses have been surprised to see how readily people of all ages who have diabetes are accepting the finger-sticks and the skills of handling the blood test strips and reading the results. The answer is that having a reliable flight plan is more fun than flying blind. This is particularly true in diabetes, which is the only disorder in which the person who has the problem has to take most of the responsibility for treatment decisions. As Dr. Lawrence Weed has said, "The greatest unused resource in health care is the mind and experience of the patient. The capacity of motivated people to solve their own problems is dynamite." You are a very important person!

The future: hope for tomorrow

Major advances in two battles against diabetes are being made. First, to treat or prevent diabetes, there must be fundamental study of its nature and causes. Basic research on insulin gene structure and expression may provide a clearer understanding of the defects in diabetes. The genes for insulin, derived from DNA technology, are being successfully introduced into diabetic tissue in animals. In answer to the question, "Why do some people get diabetes and others don't?", the role of certain viruses as an indirect cause of insulin-dependent diabetes is being studied. There may be an inherited tendency for the body's natural defenses, the immune system, to get out of control and develop an over-eager inflammatory reaction that chews up the beta cells, as well as the virus, which is the real enemy. In regard to developing non-insulin-dependent diabetes, there is a strong genetic inheritance. There are also some abnormalities, both in regard to the insulin gene and in the way in which the body releases and responds to insulin. Genetic markers for both types of diabetes may help us to identify people at risk for diabetes and prevent it.

The second battle is to improve treatment techniques and to reduce the severity of the complications of diabetes. Slow but steady progress is being made on this front also. The artificial pancreas, which can be implanted and will automatically sense the level of blood glucose and deliver insulin to control it, is still on the drawing boards. However, the so-called open-loop insulin pump is being used now by several thousand people. The open-loop pump is really a sophisticated injection system. A steady supply of background insulin is delivered automatically throughout the day, and the user activates the pump to deliver extra insulin at mealtimes or as indicated by blood tests and in case of unpredictable changes in schedule (see Chapter 12). The results have been surprisingly satisfactory. Studies show that glucose control is improved, and many people report that they feel better than they have for a long time. But, obviously, the person wearing an open-loop pump still has to be able to calculate food intake, energy output, and insulin dosage, as well as testing blood and managing a complicated instrument. The other alternative for patients with insulin-dependent diabetes who want to be in tight control of their blood glucose is to take 3 or 4 insulin injections a day (see Chapter 12). For many people this is a less costly and more flexible option, but neither option can be called a "cure."

There has long been hope and much work done in regard to transplantation of a healthy pancreas to cure diabetes, much as kidney transplants restore function to those persons whose kidneys have failed. The major obstacle to transplantation is that sooner or later the body recognizes the new tissue as foreign and rejects it through its immune system. Research is focusing on new drugs to suppress the rejection. There is also great promise in the field of transplanting insulin-producing islet cells only; this has been accomplished in animals.

As you can see, most of the progress offers more immediate hope to insulin-dependent persons than to non-insulin-dependent persons because it focuses on the pancreas. But in Type II diabetes, the problem is not so much in the pancreas as it is throughout the body's tissues where there is resistance to the actions of insulin. Fortunately, we are learning more about ways of reducing this resistance.

We have a way to go before we have a "cure." But in the meantime there is a lot we can do ourselves, right at home, with self-blood testing, our own food policies and exercise plans, and multiple injections of insulin for those who need it. A lifelong determination to stay in touch with

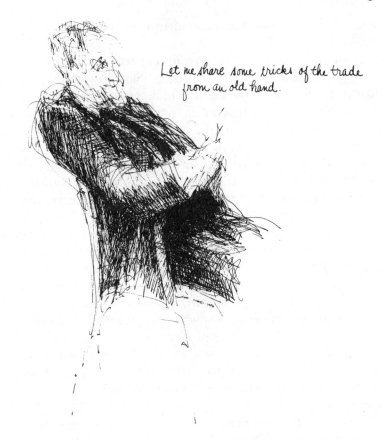

Let me share some tricks of the trade from an old hand.

up-to-date information about diabetes is another skill readily at hand. The understanding behind these skills will always be useful, and that is what this book is all about.

Tricks of the trade

We all have had the experience of having a real practical need to learn something complex and unfamiliar that we don't naturally enjoy. It may be grammar or algebra at school, the manual for the garden tractor or the stereo set at home, the language of the IRS at tax time or the stock market. Usually, we have to gear up several times, but eventually, if the reward is great enough, we put our best effort to the job and finally master the essential know-how.

Learning about how the body functions is almost like tackling three or four of those topics at once. There is a new vocabulary to learn, new ideas to grasp concerning how to calculate energy as it goes in and out of the body, and for those who take insulin, there's learning quickly how to handle some special equipment. That's a large order, especially when you didn't bargain for it. In addition, the subject at hand is one of the most complex in the world. For example, the various mechanisms by which the body keeps itself at the right temperature and able to perform under many different conditions make our most advanced computers or the instrumentation for a satellite look simple. So you're going to have to do some studying! But the reward is the greatest: *your health and happiness!* To get yourself further in tune with the positive approach to diabetes, we recommend that you also read *The Diabetic's Total Health Book* by June Biermann and Barbara Toohey. (See Appendix A.) Its main headings are "A Strong Body," "A Tranquil Mind," and "A Blithe Spirit." Although this book is not a complete manual with instructions for insulin injection and sick day management, it speaks from profound, yet humorous personal experience strengthened by good scientific understanding. It will make your adjustment easier. The goal is to look beyond survival to a balanced, satisfying life.

Here are some tricks of the trade.

From the beginning

1. Count your assets. Everyone has some, in friends and family, talents and hopes, good health aside from diabetes.
2. Think of yourself as a person with diabetes, not as a patient.
3. Make friends with your health care people. Be an equal, responsible partner in the decisions about your care.
4. Get clear in your mind which type of diabetes you have, then find out what your options are.
5. While you are developing a life plan that includes diabetes, include your family right away. Let everyone hear what the daily jobs amount to, learn emergency techniques, and decide on responsibilities.
6. Get in the habit of asking questions. Ask your doctor to share your health record with you. Ask for a short summary of it that you can carry with you when you travel.
7. Don't let anyone frighten you or make you feel guilty if you are doing your part.
8. Get in touch with a source of further education. Plan to go on learning so that you'll be up to date on the latest methods and be able to change during the different stages of your life.
9. Be yourself about your diabetes. Share this fact about you openly with others. It is not something to be ashamed of. On the con-

trary, if you are leading a full life in spite of a handicap, *you have something to offer to others!* Today, we are all more open with each other. We all move around so fast that it is easy to get left out if we don't understand each other's needs.

It is a great safety factor and a comfort for friends, school-mates, teachers, coaches, employers, fellow workers, even police, bus drivers, and airplane attendants to know that you have diabetes. They will all be glad to help you. We all need help at many points in our lives. In this spirit, get yourself an identification tag from Medic Alert, Turlock, California. Wear it with satisfaction!

10. Do not think of yourself as having an incurable disease. Think of diabetes as a correctable deficiency, which you can manage yourself. Living with diabetes means making decisions and choices. For that skill, you have to allow time to receive and manage information every day. As you know, it takes time and practice to learn a new skill. *Be good to yourself and allow time!*

When you have become skilled in self-care, your routines should not take more than half an hour a day, even if you take several insulin injections each day. However, you will also need to keep mental track of your diabetes all day and sometimes even at night. It is like the alertness you use as a good driver, which is based on really knowing how to manage your car at a reflex level in a moment of sudden change. Here are the three kinds of "time" you will need.

   a. *Time to learn how your body works:* a *lot* in the beginning, the same as for learning a new job or recipe or sport, or to find your way around a new town.

   b. *Time to manage each day,* to be master of your fate: a *little* once you have become expert, to keep your supplies handy, to figure out the special decisions for that day, to stay in touch with the signals your body sends you.

   c. *Special times: some extra,* with your health care friends, unpredictable as to when or how long. You need these special times to celebrate your successes in self-care, to renew your courage and patience, to tackle a new project or a different stage in your life.

11. When you feel truly experienced, share your skills with others. Diabetes clubs, parents' groups, and youth groups need to be formed in many communities. Members can help each other and be a great resource to the public.

12. *Don't blame all your troubles on your diabetes!* For example, some-

times it will be hard to tell at first whether you are angry, frightened, coming down with a cold, or uncomfortable because of a high or a low blood sugar level. Of course, the other side of that coin is that sometimes your family may think you are being unreasonable and cross and you may just have a low blood sugar level. Experience and patience will help you to tell which is which.

13. *Know how to reach for help if you need it.*

Chapter 2
Food is central to life

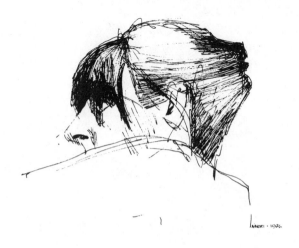

You can't eat a month's food for breakfast and I can't learn all this stuff in one week!

Develop your personal eating-exercise policy (PEEP)

Food is not only a necessity because we must eat to live; it is also central to everyone's daily experience as a source of interest and pleasure in itself and as a way to bring people together to share and celebrate. For people who have diabetes, the word diet has been closely connected with feelings of being deprived and regulated. Too much emphasis has been placed on avoiding sugars and fats and on eating carefully calculated amounts of food at the same time every day, an almost impossible assignment for anyone trying to lead a productive life in the 1980s. Much of the burden of guilt and fear among people with diabetes is food-related, and it is only now that we realize that there are other ways to approach the questions of nutrition.

One step each of us can take, diabetic or not, is to be responsible for developing a Personal Eating-Exercise Policy (PEEP). This idea got its start from a recent article in *Health,* in which Dr. Theodore Van Itallie stated*:

> One can look at meal planning as developing a Personal Eating Policy, PEP. If you find the idea of a personal eating policy strange, it's probably because you don't usually think of your behavior as being guided by a policy. Yet, it often is. You don't have to work out the pros and cons of brushing your teeth every night, for example; you already have a policy that says you do. You don't have to worry over whether or not you should toss the garbage out the window; you have a policy that says you don't. So, why not a policy to guide your food choices as well, choices that most affect the quality and length of your life?

We have just expanded this idea to include exercise for people with diabetes.

It is now recognized that the diet plan must not be developed in isolation from physical activity. Like everything else in diabetes, interaction between many forces has to be taken into account. The importance of exercise in normalizing blood glucose levels and the recent availability of SBGM offer people with diabetes some new freedoms in food choices. In addition, research is breaking new ground in looking at the way the body responds to different foods once they are eaten. Even beyond that, it has only recently been recognized that the two types of diabetes require almost opposite kinds of meal planning. Type II diabetes calls for self-restraint in the amount of food, but there is little need for a rigid meal schedule. Type I diabetes calls for more predictable, regular access to meals with freedom from guilt when there is a need to eat extra to compensate for physical activity. So it is important that nutrition skills are taught as the road to liberation rather than a set of rigid rules calling for measuring or weighing every bite. Throughout this book, we stress the importance of staying touch with up-to-date information on all aspects of diabetes. Nowhere is this more important than in the field of nutrition, which is rapidly expanding.

We are unique as individuals. Some of us are compassionate, caring personalities. Others may be outgoing, energetic, and humorous. This is also true of our physical characteristics, dark hair or fair skin, short and

---

*From Itallie, T.V.: Health, March 1983.

slender, tall and husky. With this in mind, why not focus on your diet from a purely personal viewpoint? How do you go about this? It will be helpful for you to list the personal goals that you want to achieve in relation to your lifestyle and your food intake. You will find plans outlined in the chapters on non-insulin-dependent and insulin-dependent diabetes that may help you define your own goals.

Tools of the trade: the basic kit

However, you may need to become more aware of basic facts about food before you can arrive at your goals and make adjustments in your eating habits. These facts are your "tools of the trade." Obviously, everyone consumes some sort of diet, whether or not they think of it that way. But people who have diabetes soon realize that they need to know more detail than nondiabetic people do about the composition of various foods and how the body reacts to them to balance food and exercise.

Calories and food composition

We all need a variety of nutrients to be healthy. If you learn about calories and food composition, you will have the necessary background to achieve a varied but nutritionally balanced diet. *It is not a simple subject for study, and there is no doubt that you are going to need some expert help before you can become your own nutritionist.* Here's the basic vocabulary to start with.

A calorie is a unit of energy used to express the energy-producing content of foods. A calorie (Cal) is the amount of heat needed to raise the temperature of 1 kilogram [2.2 lb] of water by 1°C. Did you ever stop to think that your hand is warm because your body is releasing the sun's energy, which had been captured in the plant and animal foods you have eaten?

Calories come from three different sources of nutrients: protein, fat, and carbohydrate. Most foods contain more than one nutrient. For instance, milk contains protein, fat, and carbohydrate. Although your diet can be made up of various combinations of these nutrients, a balanced diet (for anyone, diabetic or not!) should contain:

     50% to 60% of its calories as carbohydrate (starches, sugars)
     30% to 38% of its calories as fat
     12% to 20% of its calories as protein

This balance ensures sufficient carbohydrate for energy, a safe amount of fat, and enough protein for the continuous regeneration of body pro-

Table 1. Some examples of carbohydrates, proteins, and fats

Simple carbohydrates—sugars	Complex carbohydrates—starches (some protein too)
Milk (lactose)	Wheat
Fruit (fructose, glutose, sucrose)	Rice
White sugar	Noodles, spaghetti, macaroni
Brown sugar	Cereals
Powdered sugar	Flour
Honey	Bread
Molasses	Crackers
Maple syrup	Dried beans, pas
Corn syrup	Starchy vegetables
Jellies and jams	Corn
Candy	Lima beans
	Parsnips
	Peas
	Potatoes
	Sugar and starch combined (some protein and fat too)
	Cookies
	Cake
	Pie
	Breads and muffins

Proteins

Lower fat	Higher fat
Beef, pork, lean cuts	Cheese
Poultry	Milk, whole
Fish	Processed meats
Eggs	Meats, high-fat cuts
Mixed beans and grains	
Milk, skim and low fat	
Cheese, low fat	

Fats

Saturated		Unsaturated
Animal source	*Vegetable source*	*Vegetable source*
Butter, lard, shortening	Coconut oil	Margarine
Cream	Olives	Safflower, corn, and peanut oil
Cream cheese	Olive oil	Nuts (also provide some protein)
Salt pork		Salad dressing without eggs
Bacon		

teins. The ranges allow for differences in age, body type, and work activities. Protein and carbohydrate provide the same number of calories per gram; fats are more than twice as concentrated:

            1 gram carbohydrate yields 4 calories
            1 gram fat yields 9 calories
            1 gram protein yields 4 calories

It is also important to know that alcohol yields calories (1 gram alcohol yields 7 calories). These calories must be counted in the diet, although they provide heat but no nourishment for body energy. Table 1 provides some examples of carbohydrates, proteins, and fats.

The exchange system: one tool for meal planning

There is a national effort underway to develop new nutrition guidelines that take into consideration the great variety of individual needs and the recent knowledge about how the body responds to different foods. However, for the time being, the exchange system is one practical method for learning about food composition. You will certainly need some advice from a diet counselor to help you work out a meal plan that suits your type of diabetes and your height, weight, activity, and food likes and dislikes. If you have difficulty finding a diet counselor, your local American Diabetes Association affiliate can help you. Your diet counselor should be a dietitian but could also be a nurse or physician with special expertise.

The dietary exchange lists, as published by the American Diabetes Association and the American Dietetic Association, divide foods into classes, depending on whether they contain predominantly carbohydrate, fat, protein, or a mixture, and then tell how much of one type of food has roughly the same composition and caloric content as another food in the same class. This makes it easier to choose foods, and most people soon become very familiar with the lists and choose balanced diets automatically and correctly. Table 2 gives examples of the nutrient values of some exchanges.

In the food exchange system, all the foods you might eat are listed under the "exchange lists." For example, bread, cereal, pasta, and other starchy foods will be listed under "bread exchanges," each with an appropriate serving size listed. This means that such a serving of any of those foods will have similar amounts of carbohydrate and protein. For example, your meal plan may call for 2 bread exchanges for breakfast. You may then select 2 servings of any of the items listed on the "bread exchanges." It may be 2 of the same, such as 2 pieces of toast, or it may be 1 piece of toast and 1 serving of cereal. Your diet counselor can explain this system in de-

Table 2. Nutrient values of exchanges

| Exchange group | Amount | Composition of one exchange in grams | | | |
		Carbohydrate	Protein	Fat	Calories
Milk, whole	1 cup	12	8	10	170
Milk, low fat	1 cup	12	8	5	125
Milk, nonfat	1 cup	12	8	—	80
Vegetable	½ cup	5	2	—	28
Fruit	Varies	10	—	—	40
Bread	Varies	15	2	—	68
Meat, lean	1 ounce	—	7	3	55
Meat, medium fat	1 ounce	—	7	5	73
Meat, high fat	1 ounce	—	7	8	100
Fat	1 tsp	—	—	5	45

tail and will provide you with an exchange list describing other alternatives within the food categories, such as fish or eggs in the meat exchange and pasta and beans in the bread exchange, and how to fit in different kinds of cheese. The system is flexible enough to allow for special foods from different nations and for vegetarian menus.

How do we arrive at a meal plan?

The first consideration in developing your meal plan is your personal caloric need, which is based on your age, sex, activities, and appropriate weight. To decide how many calories you should take in per day and how they should be divided, keep a diary of your activities and food intake for 3 to 5 days and show this to your diet counselor on your next visit. Include everything about your pattern of food intake and activity, being as accurate and complete as possible. If your weekends vary significantly from your weekdays, it may be helpful to include one weekend day in your food records.

From your food records, a meal plan can be developed to serve as a guideline for your own PEEP. Your diet counselor can assist you with what would be an appropriate caloric intake based on whether you need to gain or lose weight or want to maintain your current weight.

Enough exchanges are chosen from each food group to add up to the prescribed amounts of protein, fat, and carbohydrate. Usually, the number of exchanges necessary to provide the required protein is determined first because foods that are rich in protein usually have some carbohydrate and fat in them also. Then the exchanges necessary to provide the required additional amount of carbohydrate are figured. Exchanges for fruit, which is pure carbohydrate, and fat, which is pure fat, are added last. These exchanges make up the total fat, carbohydrate, and calories of the required amount. Then the total number of exchanges is divided into meals and snacks based on your insulin requirement, if appropriate, and your activities. The total amount of carbohydrate is divided into small amounts throughout the day so as not to overload your system at any given time.

Don't worry if the first meal plan you and your diet counselor work out is not satisfactory. Keep a record of how you feel about the meal plan. If your weight is normal for you, you should not be hungry all the time. If you are overweight, you may feel hungry at times, since the goal is to reduce your weight. But be sure to discuss this with your diet counselor at your next meeting.

Remember, a diabetic diet is nothing more than a well-balanced diet, with meals spaced at regular intervals to meet the special needs of an individual. Almost everything you ate before you knew you had diabetes you can eat now in moderation. And if you learn to do it properly, you can enjoy your meals secure in the knowledge that you are taking good care of all your body systems.

After you are completely familiar with the tools of the trade in nutrition, you can use SBGM to work on your own. You can test how your body responds to different kinds of food. You can actually see the interactions between food and exercise. You can make many daily adjustments to allow for changes in schedule, exercise availability, and unplanned activities. You will develop your own PEEP, tailored to meet your needs in a way that allows you to lead a life of maximum flexibility for the 1980s. The exchange lists will probably be only one of many techniques you will use to plan and judge your food intake.

These ideas are generalities about diet. Other chapters (9 and 14) in this book discuss more specific diet plans for insulin-dependent and non-insulin-dependent diabetes.

One of the most interesting challenges you face as a person with diabetes is learning to judge the quality of books and articles on food and nutrition. Public interest in nutrition has led to a large increase in the literature, and some of the materials available are not trustworthy. If you have questions about what you've heard or read, call your local American Diabetes Association affiliate or the national office and ask for advice and reliable references.

A useful list of up-to-date books on diet and nutrition (*Diet and Nutrition for People with Diabetes*) can be obtained free from the National Diabetes Information Clearinghouse, P.O. Box NDIC, Bethesda, MD 20205. The American Diabetes Association *Family Cookbook* now has two volumes and is your best reference as far as cookbooks are concerned.

Topics of special interest: sophisticated supplements to your skills

Biological responses to food

The science of nutrition is coming up with new ways of looking at foods that may change the old rules about choosing what to eat when you have diabetes. Recently, researchers have been studying the biological effects of both simple and complex carbohydrates and how they influence blood sugar. This is a different approach because, up to now, most of the dietary recommendations concerning how food affects blood sugar levels were derived only from looking at the chemical components. Attention was focused on how much and what type of carbohydrate, protein, or fat is in a particular food or meal, as opposed to how the body handles the food once it is eaten.

Now, in looking at the biological response of the body to various foods, we see that different foods containing carbohydrates have their own unique influence on blood sugar. Testing of foods such as rice, potatoes, legumes, wheat, corn, beans, pasta, glucose, fructose, sucrose, and lactose suggests that there are wide variations in biological response to complex and simple carbohydrates. *It is clear that we do not know as much as we thought we did about which foods increase blood glucose levels.* For example, potatoes may give a more rapid rise than ice cream! Is this because there is some fat in the ice cream? Scientists are trying to organize this information by comparing each food to an equivalent amount of glucose. This system is called the glycemic impact of foods. Foods will be ranked within their groups for their effect on blood glucose levels. Of course, the volume of the foods will vary. For example, ¼ cup of maple syrup would be compared to two whole potatoes for glycemic impact. You will probably be hearing more about this as another tool for managing your food.

Does this new knowledge mean that we can ignore the old advice—to limit sugars and to increase fiber foods and complex carbohydrates in the diet? *No, it is clear that the old advice is still good advice and your PEEP will always be an essential part of self-care in diabetes.* Sugars (especially sucrose) and fats must be carefully calculated. For those who have a tendency to gain weight, *calories must be counted.* However, the rules may change as research progresses, and many questions have yet to be answered. Not all foods have been tested. Further study is needed to look at blood sugar responses to different carbohydrates when they are eaten as part of an entire meal instead of just by themselves. There is still much to be learned about interactions between different foods. There are also variations in blood sugar responses according to the physical properties of the food as it is eaten—whether it is whole, ground, or in liquid form. You need to be in touch with reliable up-to-date information on a regular basis.

Meanwhile, there are many time-tested ways of thinking about food. We can make choices in relation to our physical activities with blood monitoring to back them up. The exchange system can be used to monitor total calories and balance between all the essential nutrients. Record keeping, which focuses not only on food intake but integrates it with exercise and insulin if needed, will give you a clear picture about how your diabetes and your lifestyle are affecting each other. That's what PEEP is all about.

How to purchase food for your diet

Your diet does not cost more because you are a person with diabetes. In fact, it may cost you less if you plan wisely, shop carefully, and keep in mind your needs and those of your family. Take time to plan your meals, especially in the beginning. Know how many portions and the size of the portion from each food group you need before you go shopping. Substitute but do not add to your diet.

Today, there are many convenience foods available. We sometimes need or want to use them to save time and effort, despite the considerable extra cost involved. Convenience foods now have labels telling specifically what they contain. So it is possible to fit them into your food plan. However, keep in mind that you have less control over what you eat when you choose these precooked items. This is not only true in regard to additives, such as artificial coloring and various preservatives, but also in terms of the degree of processing and refining of the natural food stuffs, which removes both fiber and vitamins. The convenience foods may also add extra salt to your diet. Remember that ingredients are listed in decreasing order of content. For instance, in tomato soup, tomatoes are found in the largest quantity, milk and spices in lesser amounts.

In general, you will find yourself more satisfied by what you eat if you choose whole grains and fresh fruits and vegetables whenever possible. This kind of food takes longer to chew and digest, providing a more even impact on blood glucose levels and good exercise for your teeth. Your taste will soon learn to be satisfied by the natural, delicate sweetness of fructose, the sugar in fruits. These habits can be learned by all members of your family to their great benefit in long-term health.

Be familiar with the words for different forms of sugar and be alert to the fact that new sources of sugars and starches (carbohydrates) are constantly being added in food preparation. For example, white grape juice (120 calories for 6 ounces) is presently being substituted for sugar in many canned fruits. Prepared meats (sandwich loaf, bologna) have added carbohydrates. However, you can find, along with the regular canned goods, fruits canned in their own juice or water (such as pineapple) or unsweetened (such as applesauce) at the regular price.

It is not necessary to buy "dietetic" foods. They cost more and if you read the labels carefully, you will see that in many the caloric content is equal to and sometimes greater than the regular counterpart. Also, most "dietetic" foods contain a sugar alcohol such as sorbitol, which is metabolized slowly by the body but ultimately increases the blood glucose level. Such foods are usually more expensive; sometimes the price is doubled. A few "dietetic" foods may add variety to your menu and add insignificant food value. Artificially sweetened gelatin, such as D'Zerta, is an example.

Store food promptly and use perishables in time for the greatest nutritional value. Fruit such as pears and oranges should be eaten within a week after purchase; lettuce and tomatoes within a few days.

As you become more familiar with the foods, you will learn how to choose and prepare the food that is the most economical and nourishing for everyone, whether or not diabetes is present.

Why fiber is important in nutrition

In recent years, there has been a great deal of interest in the fact that people in other countries of the world, such as parts of Africa, who eat unrefined foods with little meat or fat in their diet do not develop diabetes as often as Americans. There is concern at present about the need to increase fiber content in what Americans eat, although there is some controversy about how to do it.

All the plants we use for food have various types of fibers in their natural state. These fibers help the plants to grow, to heal, to be protected from damage, and to retain nutrients. In the last 30 years in the United States, the food industry, spurred on by the supermarkets and the convenience foods, have removed much of the plant fiber through processing, refining, and precooking. The husks of rice or grains are lost in white rice or white flour. The fiber content of many fruits and vegetables is lost or altered in commercially canned and frozen foods. This loss of fiber is now known to change the way in which the body is nourished. For example, the blood glucose level rises more sharply after you drink a glass of apple juice than after you eat a whole apple.

Although plant fibers are not digested as are other parts of plant foods, they are very useful, even essential, in our diet. They provide bulk, which promotes the feeling of having had plenty to eat, and they speed up the passage of food through the stomach and intestines, which improves bowel function. Certain fibers actually slow up the absorption of carbohydrates. For these reasons, levels of blood glucose after meals are lower when fiber is added to the diet. Fibers may also act directly or indirectly to lower the blood fats that may be partly responsible for heart disease.

These facts add up to several benefits of fiber for both types of diabetes. For the person with non-insulin-dependent diabetes, the extra bulk helps to cut back on calories without feeling starved. Slowing up the absorption of carbohydrates evens out blood glucose levels after meals. This avoids the high insulin response in these people, which often results in feelings of hunger a few hours after eating. For the person with insulin-dependent diabetes, slowing up the absorption of carbohydrates also helps to even out blood glucose level swings and in many instances actually lowers insulin requirements. These benefits have led to research development of special high-carbohydrate, high-fiber diets for diabetics. Some people with both types of diabetes are thriving on this diet, although it is quite a radical change of lifestyle if you go into it all the way. It calls for altering your shopping, cooking, and eating habits toward a more vegetarian fare. If you are interested in this diet, you should begin by consulting your physician. Keep in touch with research in this area.

If your present meal plan is working well for you, you can increase your fiber intake in the following ways without any major change in your lifestyle:

1. Choose whole grain breads and cereals and add dried beans, peas, lentils, and legumes to your diet.
2. Prepare your vegetables at home from fresh produce.
3. Eat whole raw fruits and vegetables whenever possible.

One great benefit of increasing fiber in what you eat is that your food budget will be lowered!

Various forms of sugar and sugar substitutes

This list of ingredients will help you identify some of the forms of sugar found on food labels. Although these sugars vary in their sweetness, they are essentially equal in calories, measure for measure. *However, they affect the blood sugar in different ways. You will learn to use them differently.*

Glucose	The basic simple sugar found in the blood, which is either absorbed from digested food or manufactured in the body from all other sugars listed below, as well as from other carbohydrates and protein.
Dextrose	Another name for glucose.
Fructose	The very sweet sugar found in fruit, juices, and honey. Recent research indicates that fructose is not associated with such a rapid high rise in blood sugar as sucrose is. (In addition, sucrose is a stimulus to a rise in triglyceride, a blood fat.) Fructose is sweeter than sucrose, so that less is needed. Many so-called no-sugar-added products are sweetened with fructose and therefore provide considerable calories. Read the labels!
Levulose	Another name for fruit sugar or fructose.
Lactose	The sugar found in milk naturally.
Maltose	A crystalline sugar formed by the breakdown of starch.
Sucrose	Table sugar, also used in cooking. Sucrose is a stimulus to a rise in triglyceride, a blood fat. Use it sparingly.
Granulated sugar	A sweet sugar (sucrose) used most often as a cooking ingredient.
Confectioner's sugar	A powdery sweet sugar (sucrose), used most often as a cooking ingredient.
Powdered sugar	Confectioner's sugar (sucrose).
Brown sugar	A soft sweet sugar (sucrose) whose crystals are covered by a film of refined hard syrup.
Corn sugar	Sugar made from the breakdown of cornstarch.
Corn syrup	A syrup containing several different sugars obtained by the partial breakdown of cornstarch.
Honey	A very sweet thick syrup made up mostly of fructose.
Invert sugar	A combination of sugars found in fruits.
Maple syrup	A syrup made by concentrating the sap of the sugar maple.
Maple sugar	A candy made from maple syrup.
Molasses	The thick, dark to light brown syrup that is separated from raw sugar in its manufacture.
Sorghum	Syrup from the sweet juice of the sorghum grain.
Dextrin	A sugar formed by the partial breakdown of starch.
Mannitol	A sugar alcohol that is metabolized in the same way as other sugars, but absorbed more slowly.
Sorbitol	A sugar alcohol. A crystalline sugar formed by the breakdown of starch. It also is metabolized and absorbed slowly, but it does raise blood glucose levels.

Many diabetics use sugar substitutes and products containing sugar substitutes, such as diet soda and fruit-flavored drinks. Three sugar substitutes that may be familiar to you are cyclamates, saccharin, and aspartame.

Cyclamates	They were used in the United States until 1970 when they were banned by the Food and Drug Administration (FDA) as a result of rat studies linking them to cancer. However, some countries such as Canada continue to use them. It is 30 times sweeter than sucrose and does not have the metallic aftertaste associated with saccharin.
Saccharin	As a noncaloric sweetener, saccharin is about 375 times sweeter than sucrose. As with cyclamates, saccharin has been under fire by the FDA as a possible cancer-causing agent. So far, the government has kept saccharin on the market, with a warning to the public that it may have cancer-producing properties.
Aspartame	This sugar substitute is relatively new to the consumer market. It is sold under the trade name NutraSweet when it is used in commercial products such as iced tea or fruit drinks. It can also be purchased as a sugar substitute called Equal, which can be added to foods. Aspartame is a sweetener made from two amino acids, which are building blocks of proteins. It is 200 times sweeter than sucrose. If you're interested in more information, Searle Company (Searle Food Resources, Inc., Subsidiary of G.D. Searle and Company, P.O. Box 1111, Skokie, IL 60076) has a handout on NutraSweet and its use for individuals with diabetes. It can be used as table sugar as is and to sweeten desserts, such as gelatins and puddings, and sauces. At this time, it cannot be used in baking.

Suggestions for the enjoyment of eating out

While you are learning about your diet and until you understand what it's all about, you may find this section helpful when eating out. When eating at a restaurant, a friend's home, or a lunchroom, bring your common sense with you so that you can follow your plan and enjoy yourself at the same time.

1. The average menu includes soup and appetizer, main dish, vegetable, breads, and desserts. Select some of your favorites and remember how many exchanges you are allowed. Use them wisely.
2. Become familiar with your usual portion size, so you will be able to judge correctly when you are eating. Ask for a small portion, or if large portions are served, don't feel that you have to eat all the food.
3. If you don't know how a dish is prepared, feel free to ask. This will help you to make a choice. While you are still learning, it is wise to choose simply prepared food and avoid rich sauces and casseroles with many ingredients.
4. If you have a problem eating out, make a note of it, and discuss it with the dietitian at your next visit.

Here are some examples of what you might order:

Appetizers: Vegetable juices, unsweetened fruit juices, clear broth, bouillon, consomme, fresh vegetables, dill pickles, fresh fruit cocktail

Salads: Vegetable or fresh fruit salads. Use a lemon wedge, vinegar, or known amount of dressing

Vegetables: Stewed, steamed, or boiled

Potatoes: Mashed, baked, boiled, or steamed

Breads: Any kind of bread sliced in the average thickness (as long as it is not sweetened or frosted), hard or soft rolls, plain muffins, biscuits, crackers, or cornbread

Meat, fish, or chicken: Roasted, baked, broiled, or boiled (Trim off extra fat.)

Eggs: Soft or hard cooked, poached, or scrambled

Fats: Butter, margarine, salad dressings, bacon, and cream, according to the fat exchanges on your meal plan

Desserts: Fresh fruit, plain ice cream, sponge or angel food cake, gelatin, or custard

Beverages: Coffee, tea, whole milk, skim milk, buttermilk, unsweetened fruit juices

Table 3 gives exchanges for various fast foods.

Text continued on p. 36.

Table 3. Fast food exchanges

	Serving size	Calories (1 serving)	Carbohydrate (gm)	Protein (gm)	Fat (gm)	Sodium (mg)	Exchanges (1 serving)
Arby's							
Roast beef sandwich	5 oz	350	32	22	15	880	2 bread, 3 med.-fat meat
Junior roast beef sandwich	3 oz	220	21	12	9	530	1½ bread, 1 med.-fat meat, 1 fat
Turkey sandwich	6 oz	410	36	24	19	1,060	2½ bread, 2½ med.-fat meat, 1 fat
Arthur Treacher's							
Fish	2 pieces	355	25	19	20	450	1½ bread, 2 med.-fat meat, 2 fat
Fish	3 pieces	533	38	29	30	675	2½ bread, 3 med.-fat meat, 3 fat
Fish sandwich	1	440	39	16	24	836	2½ bread, 1½ med.-fat meat, 3 fat
Chips	4 oz	276	35	4	13	393	2 bread, 3 fat
Cole slaw	3 oz	123	11	1	8	266	1 bread, 1 fat
Chowder	1 bowl	112	11	5	5	835	1 bread, 1 fat
Burger King							
Hamburger	3.9 oz	290	29	15	13	525	2 bread, 2 med.-fat meat
Cheeseburger	4.4 oz	350	30	18	17	730	2 bread, 2 med.-fat meat, 1 fat
Whopper	9.2 oz	630	50	26	36	990	3 bread, 3 med.-fat meat, 4 fat
Whopper Jr.	5.1 oz	370	31	15	20	560	2 bread, 2 med.-fat meat, 2 fat
French fries	2.4 oz	210	25	3	11	230	1½ bread, 2 fat
Onion rings	2.7 oz	270	29	3	16	450	2 bread, 3 fat

Dairy Queen

Single hamburger	5 oz	360	33	21	16	630	2 bread, 2 med.-fat meat, 1 fat
Hot dog	3.5 oz	280	21	11	16	830	1½ bread, 1 med.-fat meat, 2 fat
French fries (regular)	2.5 oz	200	25	2	10	115	1½ bread, 2 fat
Cone (Small)*	3 oz	140	22	3	4	45	1 bread, 1½ fruit
Chocolate Sundae (Small)*	3.7 oz	190	33	3	4	75	2 bread, 1 fat
"Dilly" Bar*	3 oz	210	21	3	13	50	1½ bread, 3 fat
"DQ" Sandwich*	2 oz	140	24	3	4	40	1½ bread, 1 fat

Kentucky Fried Chicken

Original Recipe Chicken (Edible portion)

Wing (one piece)	1.5 oz	136	4	10	9	302	1½ med.-fat meat
Drumstick	1.6 oz	117	3	12	7	207	2 lean meat
Side breast	2.4 oz	199	7	16	12	558	½ bread, 2 med.-fat meat
Thigh	3 oz	257	7	18	18	556	½ bread, 2½ med.-fat meat, 1 fat
Keel	3.3 oz	236	7	24	12	631	½ bread, 3 med.-fat meat

(Extra crispy has more fat and approx. 50 cal. extra per piece.)

Chicken breast sandwich	5.5 oz	436	34	25	23	1,093	2 bread, 3 med.-fat meat, 1½ fat
Mashed potatoes	3 oz	64	12	2	1	268	1 bread
Gravy	1 tbsp	23	1	–	2	57	½ fat
Roll	0.7 oz	61	11	2	1	118	1 bread
Cole slaw	¾ cup	121	13	1	7	225	1 bread, 1 fat
Kentucky fries	3.4 oz	184	28	3	7	174	2 bread, 1 fat

Continued.

This chart is excerpted from a more extensive version published in *Fast Food Facts*, by the Diabetes Education Center, 4959 Excelsior Blvd., Minneapolis, MN 55436. The booklet is available for $2.50 (plus 50¢ shipping) from the Center. Nutritive values supplied by company.

*For occasional use *only*, preferably before exercise.

NA = not available.

Table 3. Fast food exchanges—cont'd

	Serving size	Calories (1 serving)	Carbohydrate (gm)	Protein (gm)	Fat (gm)	Sodium (mg)	Exchanges (1 serving)
Long John Silver's							
Chicken planks	4	457	35	27	23	NA	2 bread, 3 med.-fat meat, 1½ fat
Seafood platter							
Fish	1	183	11	11	11	NA	1 bread, 1 med.-fat meat, 1 fat
Scallops	2	94	10	4	5	NA	1 bread, 1 fat
Shrimp	2	89	10	3	4	NA	1 bread, 1 fat
Hush puppies	2	102	13	2	4	NA	1 bread, 1 fat
Fryes	3 oz	288	33	4	16	NA	2 bread, 3 fat
Cole slaw	4 oz	138	16	1	8	NA	1 bread (or 3 vegetable), 1½ fat
TOTAL		894	93	25	48	NA	6 bread, 1 vegetable, 1½ med.-fat meat, 8 fat
Clams on clam dinner	5 oz	465	46	13	25	NA	3 bread, 1 med.-fat meat, 4 fat
Clam chowder	8 oz	107	15	5	3	NA	1 bread, 1 fat
McDonald's							
Hamburger	3.5 oz	255	30	12	10	520	2 bread, 1 med.-fat meat, 1 fat
Cheeseburger	4 oz	307	30	15	14	767	2 bread, 1½ med.-fat meat, 1 fat
Big Mac	7 oz	563	41	26	33	1010	3 bread, 3 med.-fat meat, 3 fat
Quarter Pounder	5.8 oz	424	33	24	22	735	2 bread, 3 med.-fat meat, 1 fat
Filet-O-Fish	4.8 oz	432	37	14	25	781	2½ bread, 1 med.-fat meat, 4 fat
Fresh fries (regular)	2.4 oz	220	26	3	12	109	2 bread, 2 fat
Egg McMuffin	4.8 oz	327	31	19	15	885	2 bread, 2 med.-fat meat, 1 fat
Scrambled eggs (1 order)	3.4 oz	180	2	13	13	205	2 med.-fat meat, 1 fat
Hash brown potatoes (1 order)	2 oz	125	14	2	7	325	1 bread, 1 fat

Pizza Hut

Thin 'N Crispy Pizza

Beef	½ 10" pizza (3 Slices)	490	51	29	19	NA	3 bread, 3 med.-fat meat, 1 fat
Pork	"	520	51	27	23	NA	3 bread, 3 med.-fat meat, 2 fat
Cheese	"	450	54	25	15	NA	3½ bread, 3 med.-fat meat
Pepperoni	"	430	45	23	17	NA	3 bread, 2½ med.-fat meat, 1 fat
Supreme	½ 10" pizza (3 Slices)	510	51	27	21	NA	3 bread, 3 med.-fat meat, 2 fat

Thick 'N Chewy Pizza

Beef	"	620	73	38	20	NA	5 bread, 4 med.-fat meat
Pork	"	640	71	36	23	NA	5 bread, 4 med.-fat meat
Cheese	"	560	71	34	14	NA	5 bread, 3 med.-fat meat
Pepperoni	"	560	68	31	18	NA	4½ bread, 3 med.-fat meat
Supreme	"	640	74	36	22	NA	5 bread, 4 med.-fat meat

Taco Bell

Beef burrito	6.5 oz	466	37	30	21	327	2½ bread, 3 med.-fat meat, 1 fat
Beefy tostada	6.5 oz	291	21	19	15	138	1½ bread, 2 med.-fat meat, 1 fat
Enchirito	7 oz	454	42	25	21	1,175	3 bread, 3 med.-fat meat, 1 fat
Taco	3 oz	186	14	15	8	79	1 bread, 2 med.-fat meat

Wendy's

Hamburger	7 oz	470	34	26	21	774	2 bread, 3 med.-fat meat, 2 fat
Cheeseburger	8.5 oz	580	34	33	34	1,085	2 bread, 4 med.-fat meat, 3 fat
French fries	4.2 oz	330	41	5	16	112	3 bread, 3 fat
Chili	8.8 oz	230	21	19	8	1,065	1½ bread, 2 lean meat

Alcoholic beverages

Throughout history, people of all parts of the world have made alcoholic beverages out of whatever grains and fruits were available in their region. Much pleasure has come from these products, but it is well known that alcohol can also be an enemy of health, even for people who do not have diabetes. Many people with diabetes decide not to take alcohol in any form. However, many others learn how to include limited amounts of alcohol with safety in their life plan. This skill is valuable for everyone.

Research is now able to tell us how the body deals with alcohol and why it is damaging if it is taken in excess.

    1. It is made from carbohydrates and, therefore, is a rich source of calories. *However, it has little nutrient value.* It provides energy but few

Table 4. How to include alcoholic beverages in your meal plan*

Item	Brand	Calories	Measure	Wt. (gm)	Exchanges
Ale, mild	Any	102	8 fl oz	240	½ bread, ½ fat
Beer (4.5% alcohol by volume)	Any	158	12 fl oz	360	1 bread, 2 fat
Brandy or cognac	Any	68	1 fl oz	30	1½ fat
Cider, fermented	Any	68	6 fl oz	180	1½ fat
Cordials: anisette, apricot brandy, Benedictine, creme de menthe, curacao	Any	79	⅔ fl oz	20	½ bread, 1 fat
Daiquiri	Any	124	3½ fl oz	100	½ bread, 2 fat
Gin, rum, scotch, vodka, whiskey	Any	135	1½ fl oz	45	3 fat
Manhattan	Any	169	3½ fl oz	100	½ bread, 3 fat
Martini	Any	135	3½ fl oz	100	3 fat
Old-fashioned	Any	181	4 fl oz	120	¼ bread, 3½ fat
Port or muscatel	Any	158	3½ fl oz	100	1 bread, 2 fat
Tom Collins					
Regular mixer	Any	192	10 fl oz	300	½ bread, 3½ fat
Artificially sweetened mixer	Any	158	10 fl oz	300	3½ fat
Sherry, dry	Any	85	2 fl oz	60	¼ bread, 1½ fat
Wine, dry table, 12% alcohol	†	85	3½ fl oz	100	¼ bread, 1½ fat

*From *Everything you always wanted to know about exchange values,* Idaho Research Foundation, University of Idaho, Moscow, Idaho 83843. With permission from the Foundation.
†Champagne, sauterne, claret, chablis, etc.

vitamins or minerals. For those who are limited to a small number of calories because they are trying to lose weight, *calories taken in alcohol will be wasted* as far as maintaining a balanced diet. They will make good nutrition harder to achieve.

2. Although alcohol is made from carbohydrates, it behaves like a fat in the body. It raises levels of blood fats and cholesterol.
3. Alcohol is broken down in the liver by two specific enzymes at a constant, unchanging rate. *While the liver is taking care of alcohol, it is prevented from making sugar.* Therefore, if the blood glucose level drops below normal, the back-up usually provided by the release of glucose from the liver is not available. *For those diabetics who take insulin, it is therefore very important not to drink when their insulin is at the peak of its action* to avoid insulin reactions.

There is good evidence that a moderate alcohol intake does not raise blood glucose levels in well-controlled diabetics. Many diabetics succeed in including some alcohol *in their meal plan* by following these simple rules. (See also Table 4.)

1. Use alcohol only when you and your doctor have agreed on how to do it.
2. Use alcohol only in moderation and when your diabetes is in good control.
3. Eat while you drink. A small glass of milk before a drink is also good protection for the stomach and the brain.
4. Alcoholic beverages vary a great deal in their caloric content. For example, beer is 10% carbohydrates. Light beer has only 96 calories. Know the caloric count for each drink. Learn how to calculate these calories and the snacks at the time of drinking and include them in your meal plan.
5. Remember that alcohol can affect your judgment. People with diabetes have a lot to do to stay active and healthy without losing their judgment.

Diabetes does not combine well with too much alcohol. The motto is: "DRINK WITHIN GUIDELINES."

Chapter 3
Fitness through physical activity and exercise

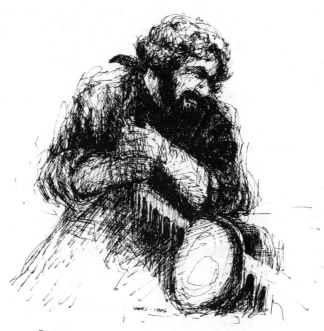

Don't call me a patient unless I'm sick!

General considerations

Physical activity is as important to every human being for long-term health and survival as food. The person with diabetes is no exception. We should always think of activity and food in relation to each other. Together they form the never-ending cycle of energy exchanges in all forms of life. In fact, there is good evidence that inactivity can kill.

Every healthy young child knows the joy of using a well-functioning body. But as we become adult, many of us lose the capacity for enjoyment of physical activity. In the not-too-distant past, people spent most of their working energies on producing and gathering food, and they worked hard. Indeed, our bodies became adapted to handle intense physical activity and also to survive recurrent periods of famine. The ability to store fat had survival value—and still has in parts of the world where food is in short supply. However, in the last 30 years, we've had our habits of eating and of exercise changed by advertising, technology, and the continual availability of food. Many of us eat more than we need and move less than we should. Today, we must all engineer activity into our daily lives. It is particularly important if you have diabetes of either type that you preserve or recapture this inborn physical capacity as part of caring for yourself.

Exercise has a strong, built-in emotional aspect. In the distant past, the ability to move fast and efficiently was closely linked to survival. You and your family won out in the hard battle for life if you got there first to capture the food. That is why people get so much satisfaction now out of competitive sports. They are survival in the form of games. Success in developing personal physical fitness does a lot for self-confidence. People who have diabetes have a harder time than nondiabetics in physical achievement. But, nonetheless, it is worth pursuing for overall health reasons. The goal is to find a variety of activities that you enjoy.

Exercise demands a coordinated response from the body's nerves and hormones to the call for extra energy. The response is directed by the brain. This communication system makes the different fuels in the body available as needed and replenishes stored fuels during and after exercise. The system is precisely tuned to meet changing demands in nondiabetic persons. Diabetic persons must plan the timing of their exercise and eating more carefully to make the most of the effort.

People vary a great deal in their personal desire for exercise, their physical need and ability to exercise, and their metabolic response to exercise. This is even truer of diabetic persons than of nondiabetic persons. Therefore, there is no one general prescription for exercise that fits everyone, any more than there is for food. It is a matter of ongoing negotiation between you and your physician. Both the goals and the patterns of activity will differ, depending on which of the two types of diabetes you have. Persons with Type I diabetes have to think for the pancreas when they exercise, adjusting insulin and food to compensate. It is not absolutely necessary that they exercise to control their diabetes. Persons with Type II diabetes, who are often overweight, do not have to worry about low blood glucose if they are not taking insulin or oral agents. But they do need a lot of determination to get going and keep going. For them, however, the payoff may be excellent control without medication and even reversal of the diabetic state.

Benefits of physical activity

Physical activity can be undertaken at many different levels, from exercises for people in wheelchairs to intense training for Olympic sports. Physical activity is for everyday, several times a day, just as food is. It is right here, available in everything we do, not just in organized sports. We do not have to spend a lot of time or money on it or wear ourselves out competing with others, unless that is something we need and enjoy. There are as many ways to improve our physical fitness as there are ways to eat. Hard exercise once a week is not enough. We don't eat just once a week! Skilled use of physical activity is one of the best ways to expand the range of pleasure in life and of improving the bargain that you have to strike with the limitation of having diabetes.

Exercise promotes good circulation by lowering blood fats and actually increasing the number of small blood vessels going to the muscles. The amount of blood that the heart can deliver at one stroke is increased. If you are well-exercised, your pulse rate will go down. Developing a circulatory system with this kind of reserve capacity is good insurance against heart trouble.

Even mild exercise helps to replace the loss of muscle mass from a sedentary life. Many people have a normal body weight by the usual weight tables, but if they have accumulated fat while their muscles wasted from inactivity, they are very much like the truly overweight person.

Exercise increases the body's ability to use oxygen and therefore to do work. Your endurance will improve in all your activities.

Exercise increases the effectiveness of insulin and the rate at which glucose is used in the body. In other words, you can burn off calories.

In all body cells, there are minute structures, the mitochondria, that are responsible for the final steps in transforming the energy in food into usable form. When you exercise, you actually increase the number of these little power plants in the body. This will raise your energy output and, therefore, make it easier for you to maintain weight with a reasonable diet.

In diabetes, exercise and diet must be thought of in relation to each other. Exercise can liberalize the diet, especially now that we have SBGM. Exercise in diabetes affects each individual differently. SBGM helps in choosing your PEEP. Discuss it with your doctor.

Exercise can help bring you happiness. Some people believe that no one can really enjoy physical exertion. Certainly, people who are not in good condition may find almost any sort of exertion a misery to start with. However, your body will reward your efforts. As you become more active, you will find you move more easily and gracefully and eventually you will recover the natural sense of pleasure in movement. If you can work through to gain your "second wind," you will experience a state of physical relaxation that persists even after the workout is over. Nowadays, people have been led to expect a pill for relief of any mild discomfort, depression, or anxiety. Exercise can be a useful, effective—and much healthier—alternative. Better to be busy than bored!

Charting and calculating energy expenditure

Figs. 1 to 4 give examples of how physical activity can be included and calculated in a normal day without costing much in terms of time or money. Of course, if you exercise vigorously, such as jogging instead of strolling, you will need less time for the activity!

It is important, especially for the person with diabetes who tends to gain weight, to recognize just what can be realistically expected as a result of daily exercise. There is no question but that it may make all the difference in the long run in maintaining the weight most appropriate for you. But it is not practical to exercise hard and often enough to compensate for eating many more calories than you need on a daily basis. For example, a piece of apple pie or strawberry shortcake containing from 380 to 400 calories would require over an hour of walking at level 4 or 15 to 30 minutes of jogging at level 6 to burn up the energy in that dessert.

A warning

If you are not in very good condition, or if you have had diabetes for many years, you should begin your exercise program gradually after con-

Examples of energy expenditure Choose your own—chart your day

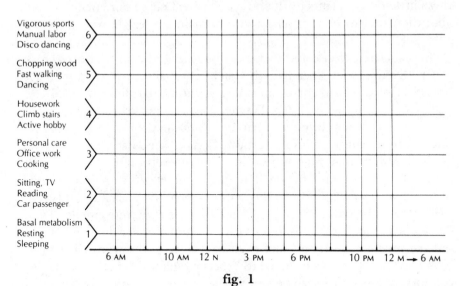

fig. 1

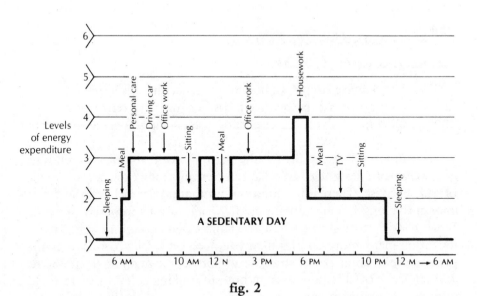

fig. 2

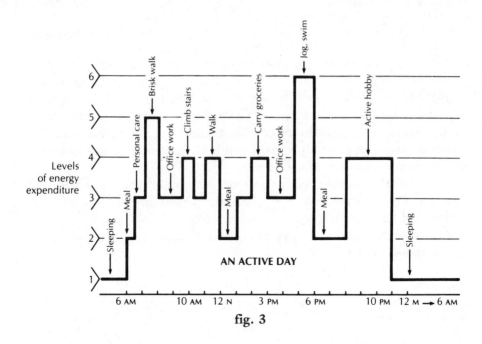

fig. 3

ESTIMATE OF CALORIC EXPENDITURE

Estimate the time in hours and decimals of hours for any given activity. List in one category only. If the activity falls between two of the grades, list part time under each to obtain an average estimate

NAME _____

MONTH _____ YEAR ____

*REF: Sports Medicine, January, 1977, p.49.

	kcal/hr	Date: _____ Hours	Daily total	Date: _____ Hours	Daily total	Date: _____ Hours	Daily total
Sleeping	70	8	560				
Dressing, shaving, showering	200	1	200				
Sitting, TV, typing, study	120	10	1200				
Walking, slowly 2.4 mph	200-250	.50	125				
Walking, fast 4.8 mph	400-600						
Walking up hill (equiv. Main St.) slowly 2.4 mph	300-350						
fast 4.8 mph	650-700						
Walking up stairs	350-750	.50	75				
Walking down stairs slowly	250-400						
Calisthenics (pushups, etc.)	150-400						
Driving car or cycle	170-200	1	200				
Jogging (estimate speed)	600-800	.50	400				
Ping pong	260						
Paddle ball	500						
Swimming	300-700						
Golf	300-500						
Tennis	400-500						
Bowling	250-400						
Light work (kcal/hr)	100-300	2.50	500				
Heavy physical work (kcal/hr)	300-600						
		24 hrs.	3260				

fig. 4

sulting your physician. Your exercise program should take into consideration the condition of your heart and your eyes. If there has been any damage to the blood vessels in your eyes, it is best to avoid the kinds of exercise that involve bending over or straining. To avoid discomfort or injury, your feet should also be checked for any evidence of faulty weight bearing. In any case, it will be worthwhile to buy good quality footwear for whatever exercise you choose.

In brief, the main benefit of exercise is not only that it can burn off unwanted calories and make you a healthier person, but you also will feel better and have an increased enjoyment of life. As you read further, remember what we said in the beginning of this chapter: always think of activity and food in relation to each other!

Chapter 4
Monitoring diabetes with blood and urine tests

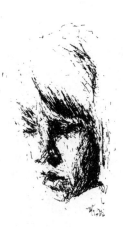

My teacher didn't use to understand why I had to go to the bathroom twice before lunch. Now I don't have to.

Reasons for monitoring blood

When you do not have enough insulin, your entire system for regulating body fuels has a communication gap. To bridge this communication gap, the person with diabetes learns to develop a mental computer system for judging how much to eat, when to exercise, and what to do about insulin if it is needed. Computers only give useful answers when you feed them the right information. The most critical information is the best possible estimate of your blood glucose level. You do not monitor your blood glucose to please the doctor or the nurse! You do not need to be ashamed or frightened if your test for blood glucose is high unless you have deliberately overeaten, underexercised, or forgotten or delayed a meal or insulin. If your tests are high a lot of the time, something must be changed in your daily plan. You will be in a position to make the right changes only if you know what's going on yourself. Above all, remember that you are the boss. To be a good boss, you need all the information you can lay your hands on to operate your energy plant. There are good tools available today. Self-blood glucose monitoring (SBGM) is an important new one. Many, both physicians and persons with diabetes of both types, say that the ability to monitor your own blood glucose levels is the greatest advance in self-care since the discovery of insulin. Why?

Remember your goals: To maximize your active participation and enjoyment in life by feeling well every day and to maximize your chances of maintaining your health for the long term by avoiding the complications of diabetes that cause so much anxiety and misery. There is no absolute guarantee that everyone can avoid all the complications. But there is more and more evidence that SBGM is the key to achieving your goals. SBGM shows us whether the treatment plan is practical and effective when it is put into effect in normal living conditions. The person with diabetes can now bring to the doctor this information, which is interesting and reliable for them both. They can then decide together how to modify the strategies of self-care, if necessary.

One of the most frustrating aspects of living with diabetes for everyone involved has been flying blind as far as knowing whether all the self-care disciplines are really paying off. Urine tests are, at best, only a second-hand index of the blood glucose, and the urine glucose is always several hours behind the blood glucose level. The kidney filters about 40 gallons of fluid a day and reabsorbs essentially all the glucose and other vital elements needed for nourishment. A normal blood glucose will vary from 60 to 110 mg during fasting and may reach from 120 to 160 mg after meals. But if the blood glucose rises above 180, the kidney is no longer able to reabsorb it all and the extra glucose appears in the urine. Glucose will persist in the urine for some hours after the blood glucose has fallen. Therefore, a negative urine glucose test only tells you that your blood glucose is somewhere below 180. *It does not tell you if it is much too low.* A positive urine glucose test only tells you that at some point since your last meal, your blood glucose was high. In addition, if your bladder has not emptied completely, some glucose from an earlier testing may still be present. Another unreliable factor in people who have had diabetes for many years may be that the kidney has developed an increased capacity to retain glucose. This means that *the urine may be apparently negative but the blood glucose may be way above normal.* Sometimes people who have no symptoms go for years with untreated diabetes. And even if they know they have diabetes, they may think that it is being well controlled when it is not, based on misleading urine glucose tests.

In addition to the security of having accurate information about your blood available to you at any time of day or night, there is the psychological satisfaction of looking at one's own test results. If they are within acceptable range, about 60 to 180 for people with diabetes, it cheers you on and motivates you with instant positive feedback. If the results are too high or too low, it teaches you to think about the reasons and motivates better decision making. When the results are not ideal, you should not interpret this as failure, but rather as a stimulus to think and discuss possible changes with your physician.

SBGM offers you greater flexibility in your daily life. It will give you the information needed to adjust food, insulin, and exercise to meet variations in your schedule or unexpected stresses such as illness, a new job, or a change in relationships. After you have learned the basic routines, you will find that blood tests can help you decide whether or not to eat your snack, delay a meal, or go for a run during coffee break. You will also be able to deal with vacation events spontaneously. It is a real quality of life tool for both types of diabetes.

What does it involve?

The techniques for testing the blood glucose, like everything else in diabetes, take some practice and cost something in time and money. Following is an introductory outline of the steps involved:

1. Ask your physician about it and find out where you can watch a demonstration. Your local American Diabetes Association affiliate, your pharmacist, or a nurse in the clinic are all good sources.
2. Buy a spring-loaded, automatic finger-stick device, such as the Autolet made by Ulster Scientific, the Autoclix made by Biodynamics, and the Monojector made by Monoject or any of a variety of newer devices. You will need a vial of test strips. Most of these companies make their own and also make a meter on which to read the test results. By the time this book is in your hands, there will probably be some new ones, so you need to go to one of the reliable, impartial sources mentioned above for up-to-date information on your options. The test strips do not have to be read on

a meter. Most people with good vision read them against the color chart on the bottle, the same way you used to do with the urine test strips. The test strips cost about 50¢ a piece. Prices vary and it pays to shop around or even order in bulk with a group.

3. Wash your hands and prick any finger or thumb, using the sides rather than the center of the pad. The blood is easier to get, and the discomfort is small.

4. Squeeze a large "hanging drop" of blood onto the test end of the strip, carefully noting the time to the second on a watch with a sweephand or a readout for seconds. The directions vary some- what from product to product, so read them carefully.

5. Wipe or wash the blood off exactly as directed by the manufacturer.

6. Read the result after the recommended time interval. You will be- come very skillful and fast and your fingers will become less sensi- tive sooner than you think.

How do you interpret the results?

Remember that even in nondiabetic persons, normal blood glucose varies from around 60 to 160. The range considered as "normal" for people with diabetes is somewhat larger because it is very difficult to mimic the pancreas with the methods we have to work with now. There- fore, if the results of your tests are between 60 and 180, you can be quite pleased. If the results are often outside that range, you should talk with your doctor about what may be causing the abnormal blood glucose in your overall treatment plan and your ability to make it work.

How should the tests be read and is it necessary to buy a meter to be accurate?

The meters will give very precise readings, such as 123 or 247. This degree of exactness is not really necessary because the blood glucose varies throughout the day in the normal course of events. However, some peo- ple prefer the meter because it avoids having to guess at the readings when the colors on the test strips are somewhere between the sample colors on the bottle. With practice, you can interpret the colors with enough accura- cy to guide your decisions, if your color vision is good. For those who wish to be very precise about blood glucose such as during pregnancy, the meters can be valuable. Many insurance policies will now pay for them, and now that there are several models, the prices are coming down some- what. Shop around to compare convenience features.

When and how often should you test?

When you decide to begin blood monitoring you will want to gather enough information throughout the day so that you know your own pattern of response to food, exercise, and insulin, if you take it. This means 3 to 4 tests a day at first, before each meal and at bedtime, at least 2 days a week. One of the days should be a weekend day because it probably is different in activities from weekdays. After you have stabilized your treatment plan, you may be able to reduce the number of tests and rely on urine tests some of the time. You will also find it reassuring to have this skill right at hand to use at odd times of the day, such as before and after exercise, or during the middle of the night if you waken with what feels like a low blood glucose. One great advantage of blood testing is that you don't have to go to the bathroom to do it! That can be a big help when you are traveling.

Why should you consider doing it if you feel satisfied the way you are?

There are several reasons for you to consider it carefully. First, you may not be doing as well as you think you are and blood testing will help you to find this out and correct it. This is especially true for persons with Type II diabetes. If your kidney has already developed an increased capacity to retain urine sugar, those urine tests are not telling you the real story. In regard to staying with your PEEP, many is the person with Type II diabetes who has been delighted to be able to see that a rapid walk after dinner or real restraint at Thanksgiving time actually pays off in a lower blood glucose level.

Second, you will find that the burdens of guilt, frustration, and anxiety will be eased when you know what you're dealing with. You may have been wasting energy on these bad feelings when it wasn't necessary at all.

Last but not least, when they come up with a cure, you want to be there to enjoy it!

Glycosylated hemoglobin (HgAlc)

Recently, a new test has become available that can measure blood glucose levels as they are averaged over the previous 3 months. Research shows that when blood glucose rises above a normal level, some glucose attaches itself to hemoglobin A in red blood cells. Then the hemoglobin is chemically changed to Alc, which can now be measured. Red blood cells last for about 100 days in the bloodstream, so the measurement indicates how effective the treatment plan has been, averaging over that period. This information adds to the data you have collected from self-monitoring. You should ask your doctor for this test 3 to 4 times a year. It will help you both.

Urine testing: is there any use for it?

Yes, indeed, it is still useful. It is an alternative and a back-up to blood testing once you have learned the pattern of your body's response to food, exercise, and medication. This is especially true if you test frequently, provided you remember its limitations as we described them earlier in this chapter. For one thing, it is less expensive, especially if you are at home and can use Clinitest tablets. But, most important, it is the only way you can test for *ketones*, which *are an early warning signal* that the diabetes is seriously out of control. Ketones are small fragments from the breakdown of fatty acids that appear in the urine when the cells of the body are not able to burn glucose for lack of insulin. The body is experiencing a form of starvation and turns to fat for nourishment. Ketones can also be a sign of too much insulin. In this situation, they first appear without glucose in the urine. The effect of too much insulin in the blood is also a form of starvation. Again, fat is broken down to be burned when the reserves of glucose are exhausted. For example, a 1 + or 2 + test for ketones in an early morning urine test with no glucose is proof positive that there has been an insulin reaction in the early hours of the morning.

Collecting urine to test for both types of diabetes

If you do not take insulin injections and your routine has been working well, your physician may only ask you to test the first urine after your largest meal, several times a week. If these tests are consistently positive, you probably need to make some changes in your food and exercise plans.

If your physician wishes you to check second-voided urines, please read the following paragraphs. It is helpful to understand this technique in any case, since you will find it useful in case of illness.

Second-voided urines

With the best of regulation and even in normal people, a brief spill of glucose in the urine occurs during or just after a meal. For this reason, the urine collection is usually made 3 to 4 hours after a meal. To give the most accurate, up-to-the-minute indication of blood glucose levels at that time, a collection of fresh urine is needed. To do this, the bladder should first be emptied completely. You may save this for testing in case you are unable to obtain a second voiding. In 15 or 20 minutes, a second collection is made and tested. It is called "second-voided urine," and in practice, this means planning to void twice for each urine test. Admittedly, this is a nuisance. But if, for example, all the urine that has been in the bladder overnight is tested, the glucose in the urine could reflect a high blood sugar level that occurred right after the evening meal. If you take insulin injections, you would not know if the insulin you took to cover the night was enough to do the job. So, in the long run, it pays to test the second urine. With practice, it becomes second nature.

Tools for testing for glucose

The following materials can be bought at your pharmacy without a prescription. Read the package inserts carefully to avoid misleading results and check with your nurse or physician to be sure you understand the directions.

Clinitest tablets

Clinitest tablets give the most accurate and least expensive estimate in terms of percent of sugar in the urine, but are more cumbersome than other methods. Urine is measured with a dropper into a test tube and is diluted with water. The tablet is added and allowed to dissolve and bubble. Two drops of urine to 10 drops of water gives the most sensitive and quantitative test. (Be sure to use the correct color chart. A different one is used when the test is made with 5 drops of urine.) These tablets are particularly useful in checking the total amount of glucose in a 24-hour collection. The tablets are corrosive and should be kept away from children. They should be protected against moisture; keep the bottle tightly closed.

Test tapes and "stix"

Test tapes and "stix" are convenient to use, since they need only be moistened with urine and read after a designated interval. Since the main reason for urine testing today is to keep track of ketones when you are ill or under stress, the most useful products are those that give results for both glucose and ketones. Biodynamics makes a Chemstrip UGK. Ames Company makes Ketodiastix, which also has tests for both glucose and ketones. All of these items are useful for a quick test, especially when you are traveling. But they are reliable only when fresh. Check these tapes occasionally against a urine tested by Clinitest tablets as well.

Tools for testing for ketones (acetone)

Acetest tablets (Ames Company) give a quantitative estimate of one of the ketone bodies (acetoacetate) in the urine. The tablet should be placed on a clean dry surface (not on a paper towel, which may give a false positive result) and a small drop of urine added. Note the color at exactly 15 seconds and compare it with the color chart provided. Ignore a faint blue color.

Ketostix (Ames Company) are dipsticks and may simply be dipped in a stream of urine and read after several seconds.

Check with your pharmacist to find out about new products as they become available. Shop around for the best price and consider ordering in bulk.

Chapter 5
Living with diabetes

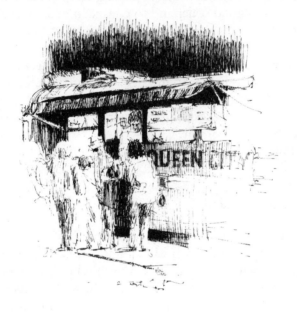

How can I ever go out to eat
or travel further than downtown?

Save your soles

The foot is a remarkable engineering design, flexible yet strong, built to last a lifetime. It is made up of 26 bones, bound together by many muscles, ligaments, and tendons that are, weight-for-weight, stronger than steel. It is nourished by a network of large and small blood vessels, in which the blood is under enough pressure to return efficiently to the heart and lungs. It is connected to the brain by long nerve cells, which relay continuous information about balance, direction, speed of motion, and possible sources of injury. In the time it takes to walk across the room, your foot will have borne a ton of weight. Food, oxygen, and information about our environment travel long distances because our feet are farthest from the supply centers of heart and brain. For this reason, injury or infection are slower to heal than in other parts of the body. This is especially true for older people, whose circulation may be less efficient as a natural part of aging.

It is easy to forget our feet, to take them for granted. Especially in northern industrialized countries, we cover our feet from daily sight and are not totally dependent on them to move us from place to place. But they are vital to health and mobility, enabling us to exercise to keep our circulatory system in good order and to engage in many forms of recreation and work.

It is especially important for persons who have diabetes to appreciate and care for their feet, to keep them clean and well protected. Injury and infection make diabetes harder to manage, and the diabetes prolongs the healing process. Most important, persons who have had diabetes for a long time may have much less acute feeling in the feet. Injury can then occur without their knowing it.

You will find some helpful suggestions to prevent foot trouble in Chapters 10 (Type II) and 15 (Type I).

Behold, the mouth!

What an important and interesting part of our bodies is the mouth! It grows to match our need for nourishment and self-expression. Eating is only a small part of what goes on in the mouth. Our lips smile or grimace as we recognize friends or enemies. Our speech, which puts us in touch with the rest of the human world for learning, for loving, for work of all kinds, is shaped by the mouth and the way the tongue hits the teeth and palate to pronounce the sounds of our language. Our mouths are part of the special beauty of each one of us, and, as we mature, the lines around it tell the tale of our adjustment to life itself.

The newborn has no teeth, since it feeds from the breast or bottle. When the baby is ready for coarser foods, 20 small teeth begin to develop. In turn, these teeth are replaced by 32 larger ones, which, if cared for and given the right kind of exercise, will last a lifetime.

The teeth are firmly rooted in the jawbones and surrounded by the gums, which come up around the sensitive neck and protect them from damage and decay. The bulk of the teeth consists of dentin. The crown, which is the part of the teeth that we can see, is covered by enamel, hard and smooth and resistant to decay. The whole system is designed to withstand 200 to 300 pounds of pressure per square inch every time we chew. That's excellent engineering to last a lifetime. Dentures can only absorb one tenth of that pressure.

The materials from which the teeth are formed depend on our diet as well as on inherited characteristics. Beginning with the diet of the mother during pregnancy, all the way to the end of life, the quality of nutrition is the most important factor. Some of the foods we eat in the United States today are not at all like the food our teeth were designed to chew. It is often lacking in fiber and is high in refined sugar. It is in childhood that habits of eating are begun. Parents can do a great service by teaching their children to avoid soft and sweet foods such as soda pop, bubble gum, and sticky, sugar-coated cereals. We can deliberately choose to buy foods that require more biting and grinding action in the mouth, such as whole grain cereals and breads, lean meat, and raw fruits and vegetables. Even a simple choice like eating a fresh apple can go far to clean the teeth after a meal, especially in contrast to a fudge brownie or a lollipop.

When we begin to eat by putting something in our mouths to chew, all sorts of signals trigger the responses of the body to receiving food and using it for energy. Digestion itself starts in the mouth with saliva, secreted from small glands under the tongue and at the back of the cheeks. The release of insulin begins as soon as we sit down to eat.

To keep the mouth healthy, we need to consider the gums around the teeth as well as the teeth themselves. Unless the teeth and gums are cleaned regularly and often, there is a colorless, transparent film called plaque that develops. It is a sticky substance like flypaper, which collects bacteria. Gingivitis, commonly called pyorrhea, is the name for irritation of the gums when they surround the neck of the teeth. If the gum becomes rough and swollen, it develops crevices or pockets where more plaque builds up. This is the beginning of periodontal disease. The bacteria and plaque on the smooth and biting surfaces of the teeth change sugars in the food we eat to acid, and a vicious cycle occurs and tooth decay is produced.

The encouraging part of this story is that we can prevent it with very little effort. Use your toothbrush and dental floss. Brush the teeth with the bristles held at 45 degrees to the surface of the teeth and gum. Move the brush with a jiggling motion so that the bristles clean between the teeth and where the gum surrounds them. Don't brush across the teeth because you can harm the teeth by grooving them at the gum line. Use dental floss to finish the job. A rubber tip is also helpful to stimulate the circulation of the blood in the gums and to wipe the crevices clean.

Everyone needs to use these old and simple remedies to prevent tooth decay and gum infection, which can lead in time to loss of teeth. But, of course, people with diabetes have strong reasons to look after their teeth because chewing is the first step in good nutrition, and infection of any kind makes diabetes harder to handle. Many people who have had diabetes for a long time without realizing it find out first when they visit their dentist. The dentist will suspect diabetes if the gums are swollen, inflamed, darkened, and bleed easily and if the teeth are extra sensitive around the neck.

The time to do something about this aspect of your health is *now*, before you have any trouble, although it is never too late to begin. In fact, if your gums are bleeding or sensitive, you will be surprised how rapidly they will return to health with a little care. Three minutes twice a day, a toothbrush, and some floss can save you many hours in the dentist's chair and lots of money and also prevent future pain and disfigurement. If you combine this skill with good management of your food, you may even have fewer cavities than nondiabetics, probably because of your low or controlled free sugar intake!

If you want more information on how to care for your mouth, write to:

American Dental Association
211 East Chicago Avenue
Chicago, IL 60611

Traveling with diabetes

We travel when we go to school or to the store, as well as to more distant places for work or vacation. The following guidelines are useful every day. *The goal is to have a good time,* both on everyday work travel and on vacations. That means:

1. Feeling well and full of energy. That only happens when blood glucose is in good control, preferably between 60 and 180 most of the time. It's worth the work it takes to keep track of it.
2. Being willing to take a few risks, try something new and unpredictable.
3. Realizing that no one can be perfect at taking care of his or her diabetes all the time!
4. Getting back home safe in body and sound in mind.

Take time to consciously go through each of the following steps:

Guidelines for happy traveling for both types of diabetes

1. Avoid the "I'm deprived and different" ego trip.
2. Plan ahead and include your family in the planning.

3. Allow time for diabetes on the trip. You can never take a vacation from it.
4. Take basic supplies of medications and testing equipment in a carryall, NOT in checked luggage.
5. Have comfortable clothes, especially shoes.
6. Take a look at your feet every day. Carry Band-Aids and Vaseline.
7. Provide for emergencies with extra supplies, extra eyeglasses, personal prescriptions.
8. Learn how to substitute one kind of carbohydrate, fat, or protein with another (exchange system) so you can enjoy local specialties and variety.
9. Come to terms with the need to balance diet and exercise. Eat less if you are sedentary in planes or at conventions. Learn how to exercise even in plane or car seats and to jog in motel rooms and allow time for it.
10. Monitoring your own blood glucose is a great advance over flying blind with unreliable urine tests. It helps in correcting problems that may arise, and it rewards you when you're doing a good job. Both types of diabetics need this skill, especially when traveling.
11. Wear your Medic Alert tag at all times.
12. Ask your doctor for a short summary of your health record to carry in your wallet.
13. If you go alone, be sure someone knows where you have gone and what your plans are.
14. If you are driving a car, eat regularly, avoid alcohol, and share the driving, if possible.

Guidelines for insulin-dependent diabetes

1. Practice being brave and clever at taking insulin and even testing blood in public places, in case it is necessary in an emergency.
2. Check and replenish personal supplies daily: food, insulin, testing equipment.
3. When crossing time zones, stay on your home time schedule until arrival. Then adjust, by skipping or adding an injection. Of course, it just naturally works out that way if you are already taking multiple injections just before meals.

Guidelines for non-insulin-dependent diabetes

1. Take along a large quantity of determination to stay on the diet!
2. Be brave enough to ask for small portions, separate servings of gravy and salad dressings, club soda instead of caloric beverages.

Remember that you don't have to clean your plate if there's more there than you need.

3. Learn to enjoy the pleasure your nose can provide. The fragrance of good food can be almost as much fun as tasting it.

4. It doesn't matter if you miss a meal, especially if you've succeeded in losing enough weight to be free of all medication.

5. Practice a variety of exercises before you go so you can be active wherever you are.

Checklist for travelers

1. Food to cover delays or time zone changes
2. Identification tag
3. Insulin and syringes
4. Testing equipment for blood and urine
5. Medications and prescriptions as necessary
6. Health record and referral to health care

Inheritance in diabetes

Our understanding of the inheritance of diabetes is expanding rapidly. Statistics on inheritance are much more optimistic than in the past. However, the more we know, the more we find that there are many factors that contribute to the inheritance of each type of diabetes and that the ways in which those factors respond to environmental influences are very complex.

It is certain that diabetes runs in families, but it is becoming very obvious that lifestyle also has a lot to do with whether or not a person develops diabetes. This is a hopeful development because we can learn to manage our environments and change our habits. We do not have to feel entirely at the mercy of our inheritance.

Investigators are now quite certain that the inheritance factors are different for the two types of diabetes. However, it may be possible to inherit a mixture of the diabetes genes, so that some people can develop a combination of types of diabetes or move from one type to another. This is very important, because if we can identify people who are at risk, we can then take appropriate steps toward prevention.

We now know that non-insulin-dependent diabetes, the kind associated with weight gain and inactivity, is more than twice as likely to be inherited as insulin-dependent diabetes. The great increase, sometimes called "epidemic," in diabetes in the last 20 years is by and large of the non-insulin-dependent variety. Since this type of diabetes can be present for many years without acute signs, it may cause damage to body tissues before it is recognized. Therefore, it is all the more important to look for early warning signs.

Evidence that the trait for non-insulin-dependent diabetes may be present includes weight gain in middle life, a family history of diabetes or obesity, and for women, large babies. Research has begun to identify some genetic patterns that make some people susceptible to weight gain and resistant to their own insulin. However, this resistance is reduced with weight loss and increase in physical activity. Therefore it is really important that every member of a family in which diabetes and obesity are present learn how to eat and exercise. Even though the diabetic trait will always be present, these good habits may suppress it.

It is a relief to be able to say that insulin-dependent diabetics are much less likely to have children with diabetes than we previously thought. We are beginning to understand why. The causes of insulin-dependent diabetes are quite different. Something causes the beta cells in the pancreas to die, and there is real anatomical breakdown. There is some evidence that an inherited factor may make these cells sensitive to attack by viruses such as mumps and the Coxsackievirus. People who have this sensitivity may also have other changes in the immune response in general, which make them more likely to develop allergic reactions to their own tissues.

Before long, there may be a way to test people for some of these inherited factors. There are already well-established techniques for matching body tissues for compatibility in organ transplants. These techniques can identify different components of human leukocyte antigen (HLA) genes, which are part of the information system by which the body recognizes and resists "foreign" elements. People with the insulin-dependent trait often have certain characteristic HLA types. As more is learned through these techniques, we may be able to identify people with an unusual predisposition to both types of diabetes.

At the present time, the whole picture is so complicated that, even using the most sophisticated computers, it is not possible to predict accurately the likelihood of children of diabetic parents developing diabetes. To add to the confusion, of course, many families have one of the traits without realizing it because diabetes has been present in the human race for thousands of years. It is estimated that 25% of American families have diabetes in their background, recognized or not.

However, it is no longer "100% certain" that children of two diabetic parents will have diabetes. The outlook for normal children in general is much brighter than before, although, of course, diabetic parents may pass on the traits from generation to generation. As research progresses, the chances of protecting against the development of diabetes even when the trait is present are increasing.

Pregnancy and gestational diabetes

The new methods and modern facilities for team management of diabetic mothers and their children in special hospital centers are comforting resources to those diabetic women who choose to have a family. Today, favorable results for both mother and child can be expected in more than 90% of all pregnancies of women with diabetes. It is, however, a very special challenge at a very special time of life. It calls for careful planning between the person with diabetes, her family, and her physician. It is advisable also to collaborate with a team that specializes in managing pregnancy in women with diabetes and that is equipped with modern laboratory and hospital facilities. It is well recognized that pregnancy is a very great stress on the woman with diabetes.

There is overwhelming evidence that keeping the mother's blood glucose as normal as possible is necessary for both mother and child. This is especially true during the first 3 months, which is the time when the baby's vital organs and brain are formed. Ideally, the mother's diabetes should be well managed for a couple of months before the pregnancy begins. Then a real dedication is required to follow the food plan, monitor the blood closely, and be willing to increase the number of insulin injections per day or use an insulin pump. With the right kind of help, this can be a period in which the mother is especially eager to learn everything she can in regard to good habits of nutrition and exercise both for her own advantage and that of her baby.

Diabetes sometimes develops during pregnancy and then disappears when the pregnancy is over. It is called *gestational diabetes,* and its importance as a warning sign of a tendency toward developing diabetes in later life has only just begun to be recognized.

Just as with all the other aspects of diabetes, the mechanisms of gestational diabetes differ for the two types of diabetes. In the latter half of pregnancy, changes in glandular function make the mother's body more resistant to the action of insulin. If the mother has a tendency toward Type II diabetes, she may already be resistant to insulin. If she cannot raise her insulin output enough to overcome the added resistance to insulin of pregnancy, a temporary diabetes may develop. Mothers with gestational diabetes have been followed up for 15 years, and it now seems that nearly 70% of those who were overweight during pregnancy have actually developed diabetes. If the gestational diabetes had been recognized as a marker for diabetes, they might have been able to avoid or postpone it if they had controlled their weight and achieved a good level of physical training during the pregnancy.

Gestational diabetes also occurs in people who will develop insulin-dependent diabetes. Perhaps the stress of pregnancy on the entire nutrition of the body is too much for the pancreas, which may be in the early stages of losing beta cell function (see Chapter 11). Results of studies of these mothers show that 40% of them may later develop insulin-dependent diabetes. It is to be hoped that through research, measures can be developed to block the damage to the pancreas to prevent or postpone the development of diabetes.

Pregnancy is a period in which diabetes that is already known to exist is often accentuated. *But increased sugar in the urine does not necessarily mean diabetes.* During pregnancy, glucose appears more readily in the urine, and if the mother is nursing the baby, milk sugar (lactose) may be excreted. To find out whether there is a high blood glucose indicating diabetes, blood sugar must be measured. A complete oral glucose tolerance test may be indicated if there is a family history or any other sign of a tendency toward diabetes.

A family is a big challenge under any circumstances. Diabetes certainly complicates the situation. If there is diabetes in your family, the decision to have children of your own instead of adopting a baby is one that deserves study on your part and discussion with your physician.

Chapter 6
The complications of diabetes

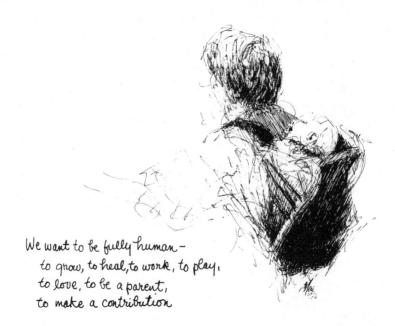

We want to be fully human —
to grow, to heal, to work, to play,
to love, to be a parent,
to make a contribution

Introduction

Throughout this book, we have emphasized feeling well and staying well by using all the tricks and tools of the trade to keep the blood glucose level as near normal as possible. The reasons are not only daily satisfaction but, more than ever before, to stand the best chance of avoiding the long-term complications of diabetes. But now that most people with diabetes are living lives of normal length, there are more people at risk than ever before. To counterbalance that fact, great advances have been made in early diagnosis and techniques of preventing and treating the problems if they do develop. Therefore, it is only sensible and honest to be up-front about these hazards so you know what you're dealing with and how to get more information if you need it.

If you are young with only a few years of insulin-dependent Type I diabetes behind you, this chapter will provide background information. It may help you make decisions about such actions as smoking. But, you should not feel burdened by daily anxiety. If you are cooperating with your self-care program and your blood tests are reasonable, your job is to develop your full potential. Of course, if you have had diabetes for many years, it pays to be more aware of what tests and protective measures you and your doctor should be taking. Following is an overall perspective on the complications.

The major complications of diabetes that threaten life itself or drastically reduce your capacity to function are all the result of damage to blood vessels, large and small. Large blood vessel disease can lead to heart disease, high blood pressure, and amputation of the legs and feet. Although people who have diabetes are more at risk for these illnesses, there is an epidemic of them in this country among the general population. There is a lot of evidence that our high-caloric, high-fat diets and sedentary daily lives contribute to this epidemic. Persons with diabetes are more at risk because their metabolism is abnormal in regard to glucose and fats. On the other hand, persons with diabetes who are taking good care of themselves are already doing everything they can to prevent large blood vessel disease. Dr. Osler said, more than 50 years ago, "One way to stay healthy is to develop a chronic disease and take good care of it!" Some people with well-managed diabetes may come out ahead of their nondiabetic friends in the long run.

We cannot predict or control many aspects of life, but smoking is a health hazard we can choose to avoid. The evidence is overwhelming that smoking is a bad influence on our bodies, not only in terms of cancer, but also in terms of large and small blood vessel function. One of the most effective health decisions we can make is not to smoke, and there are many community programs to support us in that choice.

Small blood vessel disease can lead to loss of vision and kidney failure. About 5000 people with diabetes lose their vision every year. Another 4000 need kidney dialysis. This is a very small percentage of the total number of persons with diabetes in the nation, but we need to know what to do to reduce to an absolute minimum the likelihood of these major limitations.

A secondary category of complications that may cause daily disruption because of pain and discomfort or extra time and money required in dealing with them are called neuropathies because they are caused by damage to the nervous system. There are two classes of nerves in the body. We are aware of the motor nerves that control sensation and motion. Damage to these nerves occurs quite often in the hands and feet of persons with diabetes. The other class of nerves is called the autonomic nervous system. It operates without our conscious input and controls vital organs such as the eyes, the digestive system, the sexual organs, and the bladder. Here again, there is a good deal that you can do to prevent or reverse the nerve problems. But you can readily see that uncontrolled diabetes can involve every part of the human body.

Persons with diabetes often have various skin problems, but they are generally not serious.

Diabetic ketoacidosis need not be a complication today because it can be prevented and successfully treated. It is always the result of a severe lack of insulin.

People vary a great deal in whether or not they develop complications just as they vary in their rate of aging. That variation is not well understood. Perhaps some people have inherited a susceptibility to certain kinds of circulatory damage. Many people go for very long periods without any trouble. Perhaps these people have an unknown mechanism that cleans up the debris from high blood glucose and high blood fat levels in the blood vessels and nerves.

Small blood vessel disease

The eyes

Damage to the retina of the eye is caused when the cells in the walls of the small blood vessels, the capillaries, die, resulting in leakage of fluids, hemorrhaging, swelling, and scarring. Sooner or later, most persons with diabetes show some damage to the blood vessels in the eye, but only comparatively few progress to severe retinopathy and blindness. Great advances in treatment have been made in recent years. Laser treatment can slow down the development of hemorrhages, if they are found in time. Vitrectomy can remove the jelly-like fluid in the eye, the vitreous, if it has become cloudy. Scar tissue can also be removed. Results of these treatments are improving all the time, and so is the network of community resources to help you if your vision becomes limited. Your American Diabetes Association affiliate is the best guide to these resources, and state departments of health are also an excellent source of information.

What you can do to prevent loss of vision

High blood pressure (hypertension) is often associated with damage to the eyes and the kidneys. Smoking is a very serious risk factor and increases your chances of developing high blood pressure. You should avoid smoking and ask your doctor to keep track of your blood pressure. Fortunately, high blood pressure can usually be treated by good diet and exercise, which is already part of your treatment plan for diabetes. In addition, there are now excellent medications available.

If you have any changes in your eyesight, you should report them immediately to your doctor. In any case, you should ask to have your eyes examined regularly by someone who is skilled at looking for changes in the retina of the eye. The longer you have had diabetes, the more frequently you should have your eyes checked. If the blood vessels have developed significant hemorrhages, you should plan your exercise program to avoid bending over or straining, such as in bowling or lifting weights.

The kidneys

In the kidney, the basement membrane of the walls of the capillaries may become thickened, which interferes with the ability to move oxygen and proteins across the membrane. The blood vessels may lose their filtering capacity and leak protein, which is needed in the body. If the kidney vessels become scarred, they are unable to dispose of waste products in the body.

Treatment for kidney failure includes dialysis and transplantation of a normal donor kidney. These treatments are becoming more effective, but they are very drastic. It is better to do everything you can to prevent the need for them.

What you can do to prevent kidney failure

Again, control of blood glucose appears to prevent and even reverse kidney failure and has been proved to be effective in animals. High blood pressure increases your chances of damaging your kidneys, and smoking increases your chances of developing high blood pressure. Also, you will have to face a much more restricted diet if you develop high blood pressure.

If you have repeated infections of the bladder, you should report this fact to your doctor and learn how to prevent the infections. Your doctor will want to check your urine for infection and to be sure that there is no protein leakage from the kidney. Bladder infections must be treated for at least a week with the appropriate drug. Personal hygiene after bowel movements and urination help to reduce the number of infections in women.

Large blood vessel disease

In diabetes of long-standing, the large blood vessels that serve the heart, the legs, and the feet may become clogged with blood fats so that the vessel walls become weak and scarred. When these blood vessels are damaged, the heart must work harder to pump the blood. Blood pressure rises, the heart is stressed, and circulation is less effective in bringing nutrients to all parts of the body and removing waste products. If the capillaries are also damaged, they can contribute to the damage to the large blood vessels. They bridge the gap between the big arteries carrying blood to the various parts of the body and the big veins that carry the blood back to the heart. Coronary artery disease is a result of the heart's arteries themselves being damaged.

The feet and legs are particularly at risk because they are farthest from the heart's action. When circulation of the blood is inefficient, injuries and infections may not heal, normal tissues break down, and amputations may become necessary. Peripheral vascular disease is the name of this complication of diabetes. When it is combined with neuropathy, or damage to the nerves that send messages about pain and discomfort resulting from injury or infection, the risks increase.

What you can do to prevent large blood vessel disease

Good nutrition is very important because then you can control the blood fats and glucose. Avoid high cholesterol foods and saturated fats (see Chapter 2). Ask your doctor to keep track of your blood fats. Keep up your regular exercise so that the vessels are kept clear of fats and the blood is well oxygenated. Keep to a moderate intake of alcohol and stay away from tobacco.

Loss of function and sensation resulting from neuropathy

Almost all the nerves of the body may be at risk of being damaged by the abnormal metabolism caused by diabetes. Special cells are scattered through the nerve fibers that are particularly sensitive to changes in body chemistry. The nerves are essential links in the communication system of the body that tells us about injury, illness, and danger, as well as controlling the daily function of many organs. All in all, most persons who have diabetes eventually have some type of neuropathy. The most common neuropathy is in the feet, producing uncomfortable sensations of tingling, coldness, numbness, and sometimes pain. Some diabetic persons have the same symptoms in their hands. However, many treatments are now available to slow down the damage and even reverse it and to ease the discomforts and restore function.

What you can do to prevent neuropathies

Work on your blood glucose level as regularly as sunrise and sunset! If you develop any symptoms of nerve damage, tell your doctor right away. New tests can determine how effective the circulation of the blood is and the speed with which impulses are conducted along the nerves. If you have been under stress and are having difficulty keeping your blood glucose level under control, your neuropathy may be reduced if you get back on the track again.

As far as your feet are concerned, you have the responsibility to look carefully at your feet regularly to be sure of noticing any injury or infection quickly. Your doctor should look at your feet regularly, too, to test sensation and pulses. (See Chapters 5, 10, and 15 for foot care.)

As far as your bladder is concerned, it is important to empty the bladder completely when you void to prevent infection and to get the most reliable urine for testing. It is a good habit for anyone to develop.

There is a great deal of concern in regard to impotence in men who are diabetic. There has been so much publicity about it that a good deal of poor sexual function may simply be the result of anxiety! It is very important to discuss any worry you may have in this regard with your health care team because there are now tests that can be done to determine the nature and extent of the problem and there are at least two surgical procedures that can offer relief.

Diabetic ketoacidosis

People who have diabetes are at risk for diabetic ketoacidosis (DKA) if they are sick, injured, or otherwise severely stressed. DKA occurs most often in children and young persons who may not recognize their need for extra insulin when they are ill. Another cause of DKA is failure to take insulin for a significant period, such as 1 or 2 days.

If DKA is not recognized and treated promptly, it can lead to coma and death. The body cannot tolerate such high levels of blood glucose and the ketones that accumulate when fat is broken down under such a drastic lack of insulin.

Another form of diabetic coma, hyperosmolar coma, is very dangerous for older persons with Type II diabetes. They may gradually develop a lack of insulin that is not recognized as such unless they are in touch with their doctor on a regular basis and especially when they do not feel well.

The "coma" from hypoglycemia is really a temporary unconsciousness and develops because of an extremely low blood glucose level. It is easily treated by providing glucose and by using glucagon (see Chapter 14).

Coma and death from DKA only happen rarely in this country now that medical personnel have been trained to look for diabetes in emergency rooms. The main responsibility for preventing it is yours. Wear your ID at all times in case of accident. Keep track of your blood glucose every day. Report illness to your doctor promptly. (See Chapters 10 and 15 for sick day guidelines.)

Skin problems

People with diabetes sometimes have unusually dry skin, especially if the blood glucose level is not maintained within the normal range. Sometimes, small "shinspots" appear on the legs. Some persons also develop areas of dimpling and discoloration under the skin, usually on the lower legs. These conditions are not dangerous and may disappear gradually.

As you can see, the overall message repeats itself again: Take good care of yourself!

Chapter 7
Diabetes, the family, and emotional stress

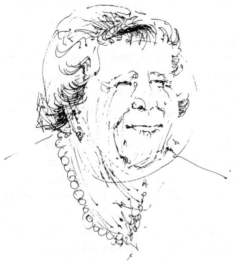

Let's not confuse ourselves by feeling guilty when we're not!

Diabetes is a special challenge to the emotions. It takes a lot of patience, a willingness to be open and flexible, and some very durable courage to live with diabetes. It takes a mind willing to be curious about how things work and a personality capable of living with uncertainty, working with questions to which there are no very good answers. Most people acquire these skills gradually as life goes on. But persons with diabetes and their families have to come up with communications skills instantly that normally take years of trial and error and forgiveness to develop. After all, diabetes makes a big dent in a family's budget of time, attention, and money. It affects everyone.

Probably the most common cause of all emotional stress is the sense of being unfairly limited by forces beyond our control. For two reasons, diabetes is certainly one of the most difficult of those limitations. First, with the limits of our know-how, no one ever completely recovers from diabetes and the daily routines of care interfere with freedom in very personal ways. Second, when a person feels ill, it's harder to be happy. In addition, it is well known that emotional stress alters the way hormones function in the body. This makes diabetes harder to control, so both those who have diabetes and those who care for persons with diabetes have to work with a lot of difficult feelings to arrive at a good team effort. This chapter on the emotions, even more than all the rest of this book, especially emphasizes the team approach. In it we will talk openly about feeling scared and frustrated as well as the times when success in care brings hope and joy.

People with diabetes and their families, doctors, nurses, and dietitians all experience all these feelings. If we look at problems and solutions together, we may develop some new and more satisfying relationships as we deal creatively with this health problem that doesn't go away.

For many years, research has rightly focused on finding out how the body functions. In more recent years, a great deal of effort has also been made to understand how people deal with all sorts of psychological difficulties, from short-term crises to problems like diabetes, which last for the rest of a person's life. It helps to know that it is okay to feel shocked, frightened, angry, and confused and that many people have survived these natural reactions and gone on to have satisfying and productive lives. Now it is important to put these two types of knowledge together. Only then can we all begin to tell the difference between physical illness and emotional stress and recognize that they can affect each other. Only then can we decide together which discomforts have to be accepted and how to reach for that acceptance in a positive way. Once that has happened, we can decide clearly what to do about those discomforts that can actually be relieved.

People who have diabetes are bound to have more than their share of both physical and emotional problems. Diabetes intensifies the human struggle because it is, in itself, a stress. Unlike the other complications of diabetes, emotional stress begins right at the beginning. But doctors, nurses, and dietitians are human beings too. Sometimes they run out of the special kind of time and patience called for in treating an ever-present health problem. This is particularly true because their training has emphasized cure and prevention and neither of these is yet fully available for diabetes.

People with diabetes know that health workers are short of time. Much of the time they do have together by appointment is understandably spent on the mechanical details of trying to keep blood glucose as normal as possible. What do the tests show? How many insulin reactions have there been and at what times of day? Has the diet and exercise plan been followed? Nobody has time or courage to come out with feelings! For example, a doctor may have good reason to be concerned about preserving the kidney function of a teenage girl. He energetically supports her taking insulin three times a day before each meal. She seems uncooperative. However, if she has been given time in the right atmosphere to describe her situation clearly, the doctor may find that she has only 12 minutes for lunch at school, including time to and from class. She does not want to lose any of that time with her friends. At this point, both the doctor and the teenager have strong feelings. Unless all these feelings come out into the open, these two people may not be able to work well together on a problem that interests them both very much indeed.

People with diabetes often have a lonely struggle because they can't get together with people like themselves. It's a great comfort to discover that someone else has had exactly the same frustration that they are experiencing. This is particularly true if they have found a practical solution to a problem that might never come up at all with the health care team.

People with diabetes and their families need to find out what is reasonable to expect from themselves and also what their responsibilities are going to be. They also need to know what they have a right to ask for in the way of support and information. To give everyone some perspective on both the trials and the benefits of coping with this particular health problem, a collection of true-to-life statements from people who live with diabetes is presented here. The statements come from people with both non-insulin-dependent and insulin-dependent diabetes. Emotional stress is not limited to youth and their parents or just to those who take insulin. So, the first order of business is always to know which type of diabetes is involved. The way the emotional hassles show up is different, although the underlying elements of fear and frustration are the same.

A quick glance at this next section will show that there are more examples of stress in insulin-dependent diabetes than from non-insulin-dependent people. Why, since 85% to 90% of diabetes in the United States occurs in people who have gained weight but still produce insulin? There are two reasons. First, the person who takes insulin injections runs greater risks every day from extremes of low or high blood glucose levels.

These people also have many more daily care tasks to perform. Since their needs are special, the opportunities for poor adaptation and conflicts are greater. Second, more is known about the underlying mechanisms of insulin-dependent diabetes. Both types call for changes in lifestyle, but non-insulin-dependent diabetes is still somewhat a mystery. We know that some people need to eat a lot less than others to stay healthy. Perhaps the same hereditary factors that produce diabetes also produce a strong tendency to gain weight. But even if we had an artificial pancreas tomorrow, their needs would not be met, because more insulin may only make these people worse. Much more research needs to be done to understand these problems and how to treat them effectively and sympathetically. In the meantime, for people who are overweight, stress comes in just one form, the frustration of trying to follow a program of diet and exercise that does not always work. These people command our respect and support.

What bothers you most about living with diabetes?

People with non-insulin-dependent diabetes speak

"The worst thing for me used to be being blamed for my diabetes when I was quite overweight. If you take insulin, at least you're not blamed for the diabetes! But people who are overweight have a hard time in our society in lots of ways. Now that I have lost weight, the worst thing for me is trying not to think about food I can't eat when I have to cook it for my healthy, hungry family every day, all year long," said Edith, 40 years old and mother of five. "Our family has been really great and we've all changed our food habits a great deal. But I'm simply wiped out for the rest of my life as far as eating whenever and whatever I want. That's not fair and it's not easy."

It's true that Edith did nothing to deserve her problem. It's even truer that dealing with her particular type of diabetes is not easy. We are finally recognizing that overcoming a tendency to diabetes and obesity is a very serious lifelong challenge. It calls for just as much study, caring, decision making, restraint, and courage as it does to manage insulin-dependent diabetes. Nothing dramatic happens when Edith fails in self-care. Nothing dramatic happens when she succeeds either! So she gets comparatively little sympathy or reward for the effort she puts in every day to keep her weight down and increase her exercise so her own insulin is effective. Perhaps the family can take over some of the cooking and the dishes so that Edith is not tempted to taste and clean up the leftovers.

Some special celebrations when Edith does a good job maintaining her health would help her to keep up her courage.

> "How can I be expected to lose weight when there is food around me all day long even at my desk," asks a 32-year-old typist. "People seem to eat 24 hours a day now, so someone is always munching nearby. There are coffee breaks and soda machines and cafeterias and candy counters in bookstores and newsstands. Eating is one of the greatest pleasures in life and I seem to spend my entire time denying myself what everyone else can enjoy."

> "When I was a child," says a 65-year-old widow, "no one went to the icebox between meals. Everything we ate was at mealtimes, which were at regular hours for us all together. We looked forward to these times, not just because we were hungry, but for family fights and fun. The food was not very varied, except by the seasons. We got excited over fresh strawberries and ripe corn. I think one reason so many of us are overweight today is that we are lonesome and bored. We tend to eat all day because food is easy to reach for."

These two people tell us how our habits as a nation have changed in the last 40 years. There is no prescription to take care of these temptations. Changing our behavior is a long process of reeducation of the self, and there are not enough people trained to know how to help us.

> "I resent having had it hidden from me that I can have more to eat if I exercise really vigorously and regularly," says a 45-year-old businessman. "Even if it's only a little more, it means that I have earned something. I have improved my bargain with diabetes. Sometimes it seems as if the health care people are determined to eliminate the pleasure principle. I need to enjoy my food like anyone else. There's too much emphasis on what's forbidden. Now I've learned to think about calories like money. You can invest them in exercise and budget for a treat once in a while."

The pleasure principle is probably more important to people with life-long limitation than to the ordinary mortal. The doctor, nurse, and dietitian who trust their clients with all available information may find them to be very cooperative. That will be a pleasure principle that works for everyone!

> "I live alone. My job is nightshift guard at a generating station. I don't have a family to come home to. It makes me angry that I'm not supposed to have beer and pizza with the other guys on the shift. What am I going to eat at the Pizza Hut?"

> "I live on a dirt road way out in the country with my four kids and my mother. My husband is a forester and he's away a lot. My

mother lost both her legs with the sugar. I'll probably get it in a few years. The visiting nurse says we shouldn't eat candy and chips when we watch the TV. But, there's not much to do and it's too cold in winter to go out. So, we enjoy ourselves inside while we can."

Here are two people for whom loneliness is complicated by diabetes in very different ways. It will not be easy to persuade either of them that they can improve their health and enjoy their lives at the same time.

Persons with insulin-dependent diabetes speak

"What I hate most is testing," says Kathie unhesitatingly, now 11 years old and having had diabetes since she was 3. "I have to remember it. I have to leave whatever we're all doing for it and write it down. When the test shows sugar, my first feeling is 'what did I do wrong?' I hate feeling guilty, especially when I'm not!"

Here is a responsible young person who is growing beautifully, doing well in school, and who has ridden 31 miles in a Bike-a-thon. But despite her most faithful efforts, Kathy can't always come up winning in self-care because the methods we have to use today to give insulin and keep track of blood glucose are not yet perfect. Her feelings of guilt and frustration need to be dealt with just as much as the insulin dosage.

"What I hate most is having to plan things," says 16-year-old John. "Every day is full of questions I can't answer. How much exercise will I have today? How long will my exam last? What will there be to eat at my friend's house and when will it be ready? Have I got all my supplies with me? Will anyone I'm with today have to wait for me? And my doctor keeps telling me I'm normal—just like everyone else! Not really!"

"What *I* hate most," says his mother, "is wondering whether he's had an insulin reaction when he goes out to run around the block after dinner and is gone 2 hours! Of course, he was just talking to his girl friend on the corner."

No one likes to feel different from friends and colleagues. Figuring out when to let one's children make their own mistakes, even if dangerous, is one of the hardest parts of being a parent. Those two stresses together are an explosive mix. Both parents and young people need special support during this period.

"It's a cop-out to excuse yourself or lean on your diabetes and it doesn't take long to learn when you're doing that," says a 30-year-old computer programmer. "But, sometimes my diabetes really does get out of control. I dislike having to tell my supervisor. However, now, when I see things slipping, I go to him first before I blow it and ask him to bear with me. I think when people use their diabetes the wrong way, it's due to a lack of basic education. They just haven't learned how to prevent insulin reactions or deal with illness."

It's hard on one's self-esteem to admit imperfection or failure, especially when job discrimination still lurks around the corner. It takes energy to plan a whole day ahead and to be willing to talk about the necessary compromises. With the best will in the world, none of that can happen unless the person with diabetes knows the reasons behind the daily routines for each of the two types of diabetes. Health professionals who are patient teachers have a great gift to give.

"What I get mad at is unpredictability no matter how hard I try," says a health worker. "No one can keep up with the world today and do exactly the same thing at the same time every day. I put good effort into regulating meals and exercise, but quite often there are big swings in blood glucose anyway. I can accept that now, with difficulty. But, I bitterly resent any implication that I am not trying. I am just absolutely sure that there's a lot going on in my body that no one understands yet. Why not say so right out?"

The feeling that you're not being told the whole story is one of the hardest burdens a person with diabetes has to face. It helps to understand the reasons why this can happen. In this particular case, there is very recent evidence that this person with diabetes may have a pancreas that not only lacks insulin but also lacks the hormone that raises blood glucose, glucagon. But sometimes the health professional has not been given time enough to be up-to-the-minute on research. Sometimes there aren't any good answers yet. Sometimes there is disagreement about which is the best answer. These difficult dilemmas for the health professional can best be solved by recognizing that it is perfectly okay to say, "I don't know yet and I'll try to find out."

"It's really tricky telling the difference between blood glucose swings and being upset," says an insulin-dependent mother. "My heart pounds and I feel shaken if I'm frightened or very angry. The same thing happens with a low blood sugar. I know it's caused by a release of adrenaline in both cases. When you combine these two feelings it can be very rough. Then, if my blood sugar goes much too high, I feel as if I were depressed, unable to act, no initiative. Which is it? Did I forget an insulin injection? It's really hard on the kids when they come home from school. I've learned a lot about being in touch with my body signals. You have to get outside yourself and try to judge the situation objectively. No one can teach that, though I get a lot of help from other diabetics. It's a very individual thing.''

Here is an example of one of the most challenging skills needed by a person with diabetes. When a crisis develops, the first task is to use the mind—to think rather than just react. That's hard enough for anyone. Now there is evidence that abnormal levels of blood glucose and insulin both affect the chemical messengers in the brain that determine our moods. That makes it even harder to think clearly.

> "When our 2-year-old daughter was first in the hospital with dia-
> betes, the nurse and the doctor, with the best intentions, tried to tell
> me more than I needed to know all at once. I remember especially the
> warning that when Cindy became adolescent, we'd all have a terrible
> time. I didn't really need to carry that anxiety at that stage along with
> all the others. Anyway, it hasn't turned out that way at all.''

Deciding how much and when to teach is like walking a tightrope for the health care team. People's ability to acquire a lot of new knowledge under stress varies all the way from not seeming to care to learn at all to being too eager to understand everything at once. In addition, it is only recently that education is recognized to be the basic need for anyone with diabetes. Nurses and doctors usually are not trained to be teachers; there has never been enough time or money allotted for that part of care. However, the situation is improving and will continue to do so, especially if those with diabetes know that they have a right to education and recognize that they also have responsibilities for their own care.

> "It's easy to mix up feeling tired and having a low blood sugar.
> It's important to figure out which it is, especially if you're in strange
> territory,'' says an active young person with diabetes. "I learned the
> hard way, *when in doubt, eat!* You can always correct a high blood
> sugar later with exercise and insulin if you guessed wrong.''

> "It's just as easy to mix up a high blood sugar with feeling tired,''
> adds a young woman who takes insulin but who also gains weight
> easily unless she exercises regularly. "One of the hardest things I do is
> to make myself run when I have a blood glucose of 220. I feel better
> within half an hour, but it's a big job to get going. I have also learned
> not to exercise if my blood glucose is over 300. It just makes matters
> worse.''

Exercise not only helps to bring a high blood sugar level down to within normal range, but it also helps the person feel more cheerful and competent. It takes a lot of cheerfulness and competence to venture far afield with diabetes, but most people feel the need to take some risks if they want to grow to their best selves. They usually find that it pays off!

> "I wish the fundraisers would tell some of the success stories of famous people with diabetes instead of terrorizing us with stories about gangrene and blindness and early death," says a 20-year-old student. "People like to support hopeful causes. It's not necessary to jerk the tears to jerk the dollars. Anyway, the place for facts about the dreaded complications is in small groups where people can ask questions and get a handle on what applies to them."

It is important to raise public awareness of diabetes because there is a real possibility that many people with diabetes and obesity in the family could avoid developing it. However, it is also important not to discourage people who already have diabetes. If they take good care of themselves, they will still be here when the artificial pancreas is available, despite all the statistics!

> "There's a lot of publicity about sexual impotence and diabetes even in nonmedical magazines these days," says a 50-year-old woman who has taken insulin for 30 years. "There's no question about it, uncontrolled diabetes can damage sexual function in both men and women. But let's not be unduly frightened. Remember that sexuality is temporarily limited for anyone just by being sick, tired, or distracted. You know, too, that if your blood sugar is out of line, you won't do well at lots of things. So don't jump to the conclusion that diabetes has ruined your sex life when things don't click. Recent studies show that a large percentage of sexual difficulty with diabetes is the result of anxiety. A healthy sex life is one of the great rewards for good daily management of diabetes. For example, when a woman keeps her diabetes in line, the urine is free of sugar. The vaginal tissues stay normal, free of burning or itching. That's a big dividend in a close relationship. Of course, if one partner has diabetes, it may take a little more patience in choosing the right times to be together. But patience is a big part of loving and it works wonders over the years. Remember, too, that sex is exercise! You may need an extra glass of juice if you take insulin injections."

Here's where an experienced person with diabetes can offer help and reassurance to others about matters that may never be discussed with the nurse or doctor.

> "You hear a lot about the effect of stress on the regulation of diabetes," says a 41-year-old contractor. "It's my opinion that, like everything else with diabetes, there's a lot of individual variation. You have to take into account the temperament of the person and the

kind of work he does as well as the type of stress. There's no doubt
that if you're sick or injured, you usually need more insulin. That will
also be true when there's a real disaster such as the loss of wife or
child or a very severe anxiety. Under such circumstances, you may not
have the energy or the opportunity to exercise as much as usual, either. However, some kinds of positive stress, such as a new job, may
call for lowering the insulin and having extra food around. Some people respond to excitement by using their bodies more actively."

Right! We all have to learn how our own bodies respond to stress.
However, severe emotional stress does affect diabetes because the body's
natural reaction to threat is to raise the blood sugar level by the release of
glycogen from the liver. In addition, if a person is grieving, it is hard to
maintain regular habits of eating and exercise. Such periods in life may
call for special help from family and health professionals and adjustments
in insulin dosage.

"When my child developed diabetes, I remember wishing it were
not my side of the family with diabetic relatives," says a young mother. "I know now that it didn't make any sense to feel guilty personally. But I did, and I never asked anyone about it. That was foolish."

Health professionals should work well with the whole family from the
moment diabetes is diagnosed. Then they can be alert to the needs of all
family members in addition to the person with diabetes. Feeling guilty
for the wrong reason is a terrible waste of energy.

"Our 14-year-old son is giving himself and us a terrible time. He's
so angry with the world and us that he holds his diabetes over our
heads like a club. We're embarrassed to turn up in the Emergency
Room one more time. He has us over a barrel because both he and
we know that he won't make it unless we help him. Sometimes we
wonder if he takes too little or too much insulin on purpose."

Nobody wins at this game. Perhaps a couple of weeks at summer
camp would put some distance between parents and child. Everyone
would have a night's rest without interruption. Healthy companionship
with others who have diabetes and new outlets for energy would help
this young man.

However, the first question to ask is whether the boy is really angry at
the world and his family at all. Too much insulin may have been prescribed for him. His blood sugar may be swinging too low without his
realizing it. That's enough to make anyone feel angry! (See Chapter 13
regarding the Somogyi reaction.)

Has living with diabetes brought you any benefits?

"Yes, indeed," says a 43-year-old owner of his own business. "You learn not to make excuses. When there's something you don't want to do, you just say you don't want to do it. You also learn not to waste time saying 'why me' too often. Life is unfair to many besides diabetics."

"I've learned a lot about guilt. We all make mistakes, but if you do your part to the best of your ability, it's not necessary to feel guilty if things go wrong. You just try to understand what's going on and figure out how to do better next time or accept what you can't change." So says a 60-year-old woman who is gradually losing her sight after having had diabetes for 35 years.

"Fear of the complications such as kidney damage or concern as to whether to try to have a child can get to you," says a recently married 26-year-old woman. "I deal with that by keeping busy at my job and sharing as a volunteer the skills I already have in taking care of my diabetes. It's a great boost to be in touch with people working for diabetes because you can keep up with the latest developments in research."

"When our daughter developed diabetes at the age of 10," says a mother of six children, "we decided to share the planning for our food, the shopping and the cooking, and to eat breakfast and dinner together at regular times. We have all gained in experience, responsibility, and cooperation. We make decisions as a group now, so no one feels left out. We find that our family life is richer and happier than when we were each going our own way at top speed."

A health educator in her mid-thirties said, "A rigid meal schedule and urine testing can be 'The great interrupters.' I have to travel a lot. I deal with my irritation by studying about the latest developments in diabetes. That way I can look for new ways to get as much freedom as I can safely. I am willing to take some kinds of responsibilities that surprise my friends, like more than two injections of insulin daily or testing my own blood. The actual tasks are easy and quick. When you know what your blood sugar is you can move fast at work or on vacation."

"It makes me laugh to watch the rest of the world struggling to give up junk food and get in shape physically. I was sorry for myself 10 years ago, but it turns out that I've been ahead of the game," comments a 26-year-old man.

"I've learned to assert myself both at home and at work," says a 40-year-old mother and administrator. "To keep my weight down, I need to enjoy the little food I can eat in the company of others, so I don't snack alone in the kitchen. Everyone comes to dinner on time now and we are thankful for the food set before us, even if I don't get much! At work, I need extra time to go to the bathroom because I walk up several flights of stairs to the bathroom farthest from my desk. This way I get some exercise into my sitting-down job. My colleagues have begun to do the same thing."

"When Jill gets sick, I care too," says Tim, younger brother of a girl with diabetes. "My brother and I used to go off in a corner and tell each other that our parents didn't care about us as much as Jill. If I hurt myself, I used to make the most of it to get some attention. But then I could see that we all care about each other equally and that Jill's problems can be really different and worse than mine. It makes me feel better to help when things get rough for her."

"People with diabetes often seem to take a special pleasure in life. I think it's because, to survive at all, they have to think about simple daily needs that most people take for granted," says a high school guidance counselor.

"Having a son with diabetes has helped me to let go of all my children," says a nurse and mother of three. "I'd like to help other mothers sort out what are normal expressions of an adolescent's need for independence and what are emotional ups and downs because the diabetes is out of line. I finally learned that you can only do so much for someone else. The other children gained from my backing off, and we are all more tolerant of each other. Of course, I never get away from worrying about the long-term complications for Dick. But then, I have special worries about each of my children."

"I am much better at organizing my time and money than lots of people I know who don't have diabetes," says a young carpenter. "All those decisions I have to make at the subconscious level every hour also seem to help me to figure out how to do my work efficiently. I know how to enjoy myself with my friends in my own way. I have a sort of internal calculator in my head so I can match food to exercise and insulin. It's a technique of thinking I can use on other problems in life."

"I surely get tired of insulin reactions and not being able to sleep in until noon on weekends. Then I remember that my sister died of diabetes just before insulin became available and I am glad to be alive," says a 60-year-old man.

"I'd very much like to write a short paperback book to show parents that diabetes isn't a disease really," says a mother of four. "Our youngest has been diabetic for a year now. It's a different way of life, that's all—a good wholesome diet and schedule for any family. Janice is pretty well regulated now. It's quite a lot for a little one to take on, but she knows more about how she feels now than the doctors or us. We're trying very hard as a family. It takes a lot of love and pulling together to meet the heartfelt needs. It makes any family stronger and closer and, after all, that's the way it should be."

Let's try to summarize what it all adds up to

These comments give us a small glimpse of the broad panorama of individual stress associated with diabetes. It is worthy of note that people don't complain about insulin injections as such. It's the unending requirement for responsible decision making about small details of daily life that wears people down. This is especially true because of the uncertainty as to whether all that trouble is really effective in the long run. Of course, the frustration and anxiety that the person with diabetes feels is also felt by health professionals.

Every human being has to differentiate as much as possible between problems of physical health and the distress that comes from feeling isolated, bored, unappreciated, unfairly restricted, or frightened. In diabetes, mind, body, and emotions have a big effect on each other. The person with diabetes needs to be considered as a whole person with a very special problem that may, over a lifetime, call for the combined skills of nutritionists, psychologists, physical therapists, and behavior modification teachers. Of course, so far, all these specialists are available to only a few of those who need them. That places a heavy burden on doctors, nurses, and people who live with diabetes alike. Here are some Golden Rules to help us.

Golden rules

1. Confront the emotions openly. Then we can all build on the constructive ones and decide together what to do about those that hurt.
2. Since diabetes is such a complex emotional stress, the people with diabetes and their health professionals will be most likely to suc-

ceed with treatment if they like each other. If they are not comfortable together, a referral is probably a good idea.

3. The daily routines should be as simple and clear as possible. No one should have to do anything that is not necessary to that individuals' particular type and stage of diabetes.

4. Since diabetes lasts a lifetime, it is especially important to have good collaboration between the people who take care of us at different stages of life: pediatrician to internist, internist with obstetrician, and so forth.

5. People with diabetes can help each other, either one-to-one or in peer support groups. Such groups, as well as educational courses, should be available to all.

6. Both health professionals and people with diabetes will gain if they are willing to learn freely from each other.

Part II
Non-insulin-dependent Type II diabetes

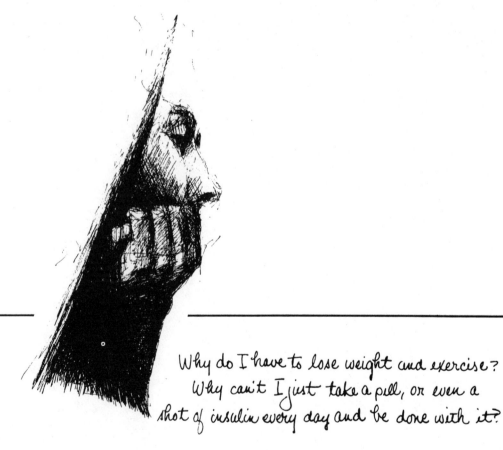

Why do I have to lose weight and exercise?
Why can't I just take a pill, or even a
shot of insulin every day and be done with it?

Chapter 8
Goals for non-insulin-dependent Type II persons

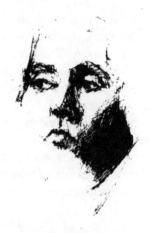

It's O.K. to tell me that no one yet knows the answers to diabetes. It helps me not to feel guilty or frightened when doctors disagree. And perhaps I can help you find some of the answers!

Learn how your body works

1. To preserve and take the best advantage of the insulin-producing capability of the beta cells in your pancreas.
2. To keep the nerves and blood vessels to all parts of the body healthy by keeping your blood glucose level as normal as possible. This will protect your heart, your brain, your sexuality, your vision, your kidneys.
3. To be active in work and recreation.

Plan

1. Extra weight is a stress on the pancreas, raising the demand for insulin. Make the most of your ability to produce insulin by achieving the weight most ideal for you. Find out what you can eat and maintain just that weight. Enjoy yourself within those limits.
2. When we exercise, we burn food more directly without calling on the pancreas for extra insulin. We keep the nerves and blood vessels healthy. We strengthen heart and lungs as well as building muscle. These physical benefits also give us a mental lift. Help yourself stay lean and lively by increasing your physical activity as much as you can every day.
3. Keep in touch with your health care team on a regular schedule so that your progress can be encouraged and you can stay up-to-date on new information about your diabetes. Join local or national diabetes associations and read *Diabetes Forecast* magazine.
4. Get a medical identification emblem and wear it at all times.

Day-to-day management: diabetes and being overweight

It's not your fault if you have Type II diabetes

As you know only too well, Type II diabetes and being overweight usually go together. But the most important research findings tell us that *gaining weight is not the result of eating too much* in people with Type II diabetes in their families. Being fat comes from a disturbance in the body's signal system about how much to eat and what to do with the calories once they are consumed. People who develop Type II diabetes have a *strongly inherited tendency* to gain weight. When weight is gained, the cells of the body resist the action of the insulin, which allows glucose to enter them to be burned for energy. Then the pancreas produces more than normal amounts of insulin to make up for this resistance. High levels of insulin in the blood encourage the further storage of calories as fat, even if the person is not eating very much. When more fat is stored and weight is gained, resistance to the actions of insulin develops in all parts of the body. It is as if you had a savings account and you put a lot of money into it, but you couldn't get it out easily. High levels of insulin may also send messages to the brain that cause an increase in appetite. Truly, a vicious cycle exists in your body that is just as demanding to live with as having no insulin of your own, as in Type I diabetes.

It is very difficult to overcome this confusion in the body's communication system with the fat cells and the brain. One thing is clear, you are not to be blamed for the problems you face. However, we are still left with the fact that a high blood glucose level is not healthy and we must do what we can to bring it back to normal. Fortunately, we are not completely at the mercy of inheritance. We can work to change our environment and our daily habits to minimize the effects of inheritance. Research is proceeding at a rapid rate to understand the decision-making patterns within the body. Perhaps a way will be developed to correct or modify the communication system between the brain and the many hormones that control the use of body fuels. But in the meantime, the best method we have at hand is diet that permits weight loss and increase in physical activity to restore sensitivity to our own insulin.

If you have been getting very little exercise and have gained weight but lost muscle strength, you may have gradually brought out into the open your inherited tendency to a high blood glucose level. But the chances are good that your diabetes does not require injected insulin for control. You probably still have lots of your own. In fact, that is why you may have been slowly developing diabetes for years without knowing it.

Recent research tells us that *you do not have to lose all the "extra weight."* It is clear that people vary a great deal in what is their normal weight. Many people with Type II diabetes have restored their blood glucose to a more normal range by losing as little as 10 pounds. Some people have replaced their weight in fat with weight in muscle and that has restored the effectiveness of their own insulin. In fact, a low-calorie diet and an increase in activity are as important in Type II diabetes as insulin is in Type I diabetes. *They are lifesaving actions that will always be a part of your daily life.* If, over the years, your insulin reserve drops too low to overcome the resistance to it or you are just unable to lose enough weight, you and your physician may decide that you also need pills or insulin injections for control. But sticking to your diet and being as active as you can will still be necessary.

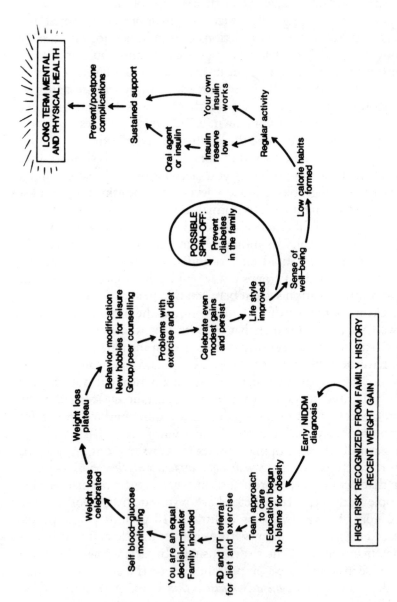

fig. 5 Spin out of the vicious cycle.
From Davidson, J.K.: *Clinical Diabetes Mellitus: a Problem-Oriented Approach*, Thieme-Stratton, Inc. (in press).

Perhaps it surprised you to learn that *you may be producing as much or more insulin than a normal person*. Why, then, are you diabetic? There are four reasons why you are in a vicious cycle, with your body systems spinning their wheels and getting you nowhere as long as you are overweight and inactive (Fig. 5). *You are resisting the action of your own insulin* in the following ways.

1. Muscle and liver cells especially resist the action of insulin in an obese person. *You can modify this resistance by exercising muscle and losing weight.*

2. One of the main actions of insulin is to *promote the storage of fat* when there is more food around than is necessary. You might think that, if you are resistant to insulin, you would not store fat. But insulin resistance does not help to keep you slim. Unfortunately, the fat cells can remain somewhat sensitive to the action of insulin even when there is greater insulin resistance in other body cells. So fat continues to be deposited. *You can reverse this factor by eating only what you need and deliberately spending calories by exercising more.*

3. In people who develop Type II diabetes, there is a *delay in the release of insulin*. Normally, insulin is continuously released from the pancreas at a slow rate except at meal times. Then, when the blood sugar starts to rise during eating, there is a quick release of additional insulin. This quickly released insulin is about five times more effective than slowly released insulin. Therefore, when there is a delay, much more insulin than normal has to be secreted to do the job. It makes you hungry and increases the storage effect. That is hard on your pancreas.

4. *The last factor is physical inactivity.* A well-exercised person has body cells that respond quickly to small amounts of insulin. Carbohydrates in food are burned easily by active muscles. Olympic athletes have low levels of insulin even though they eat a great deal. In contrast, inactive people have high levels of insulin in the blood because they have body cells that resist the action of insulin in all ways described before. *You can reverse this factor by increasing your physical activity.*

Self-rehabilitation requires support and respect

Don't let anyone tell you that breaking out of the vicious cycle will be easy. You will need just as much help, sympathy, and patience as the person who is learning to take insulin injections. You have a right to ask for that support from your family and your health care friends. There is a whole new field of behavioral medicine that is devoted to helping people make the daily decisions necessary for their health. These decisions range from the broad New Year's resolution to lose weight all the way to the small details of everyday life that make the difference in the long run. Here are some examples:

> Never eat when you are not hungry.
> Go to the grocery store *after* you've eaten, not when you're hungry.
> No second helpings.
> No dessert unless you've earned it by vigorous exercise.
> Take a walk after your biggest meal of the day.
> Get your family to take over doing the dishes so you are not tempted to clean up what they left on their plates.
> Develop some hobbies to fill leisure time.

An excellent book to help you get started is *Eating is Okay!* by Jordan, Levitz, and Kimbrell, published by Butterworth Publishers. It is a paperback.

You can *free yourself* of many of the irritations of living with diabetes. You also have the satisfaction of knowing that you are taking good care of all the body systems. As we have said before, diabetes is a disorder of overall nutrition. All the body systems get their food by being bathed in the blood that carries glucose to them. If the level of glucose is normal, the *prospects of a long and healthy life is brighter*.

Of course, even though you may bring your diabetes well under control through increased activity and diet, you may sometimes temporarily need insulin if you have an acute illness, infection, or heart attack. Insulin in these cases may be lifesaving. Please refer to Chapter 10 on testing blood and urine and sick day guidelines.

Chapter 9
More on PEEP

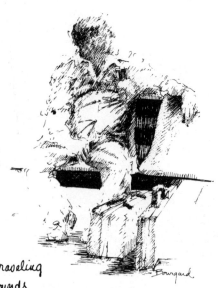

It's hard enough traveling without carrying 20 pounds extra on my body.

Physical fitness to improve insulin effectiveness

If you are overweight, your first reaction to the idea of increasing physical activity may be that you don't feel like it. There are probably two good reasons why. If you are running high blood sugars, you will not feel energetic. If you are heavier than normal for your age and height, it is simply a lot of work to move. However, let us assume that you are willing to try because you understand that exercise will help you lose weight, help you to stay leaner, and will improve your general sense of

I've just begun to eat less than I need
and I feel more energetic already. But
I'm going to need all the support I can get.

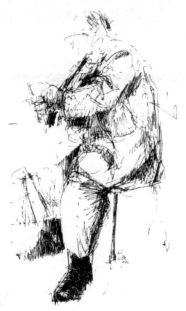

well-being. To revive your interest, please refer to the basic goals for the non-insulin-dependent diabetic and the section on exercise in Chapter 3.

To encourage yourself further, don't waste time or energy blaming your parents, your job, or yourself for being inactive and overweight. Just concentrate on finding easy natural ways to begin using your body more energetically every day.

Let's start out by asking why should "diabesity"—or diabetes closely linked with obesity—be such an outstanding feature of our Western society? Elsewhere in this book we have stressed that in industrial societies, the accent is on convenience and comfort, and our inborn mechanisms for storing energy as fat may now be responding to our disadvantage. For the first time in history, our people must make special provision for physical exertion, a fact that would seem strange to our forefathers.

Well, you can start out simply by doing your chores faster! Do things the hard way! Climb stairs instead of using elevators, walk instead of driving, carry your groceries, and work in your garden. Consider doing some mild exercise while you watch the news or, better yet, work along with one of the exercise programs on television. Do you have a friend who is a physical therapist or a dancer? He or she may be able to help you get going in the beginning and will be a cheerful admirer as you improve. You will be surprised how quickly your body will reward you! If you join a group, it will be easier and more fun to stay with it.

There are special times of life when it is easier to gain weight than others. Look at the former athlete who spreads at the waistline at age 32. What about the young mother who increases her weight a little—or a lot —with each pregnancy? These are also the most active times of life during which you can most easily lose that weight before it damages your entire body. Exercise is your best ally in this job.

One of the best ways to change your habits of physical exertion is to keep a record of your energy output every day. This will help you and your diet counselor to manage your diet in the most flexible and liberal way possible. There are many examples of record sheets and tables of caloric equivalents of various forms of exercise (see Figs. 1 to 4 in Chapter 3). Some people have found it useful to wear a pedometer, which shows how far they have walked in a day.

Don't worry that you will be hungrier after you have exercised. Contrary to popular opinion, as physical activity increases, appetite only increases little comparatively, so you come out ahead. Once you are over the hump in the beginning, you will never want to be without the daily lift that exercise provides, along with the interest in new skills and new companions that are associated with physical activities of all kinds. You will improve your health, even if your weight does not change, by replacing fat with muscle.

Even a few years ago, we felt foolish or conspicuous if we exercised in public. But now the roadsides are full of people of all ages and sizes who are running or jogging, riding bicycles, or traveling on skis. When the weather is bad, jumping rope or jogging indoors or playing indoor tennis can raise the pulse rate to 130 to 160 in a short time. Thirty minutes three times a week is a small investment of time for a great reward. Listen to the words of someone who gets a lift out of exercise.

> My exercise program gives me support even when I go off my diet. I have learned to accept myself for what I can do. I learned to get all of myself all around the track. When others flew by me in their size 10 shorts, I contented myself with my own progress. With the extra weight I was carrying, I was doing a good job. I had accomplished something! It's similar to what wheelchairbound people say when they've been able to ride a horse. They experience a sense of freedom, of doing something without restraint!

A warning

Whatever program you decide to initiate should be carefully worked out so that you feel the benefits from gradual conditioning, rather than feeling exhausted. *If you are in poor physical condition or have diabetes of long-standing, you should undertake strenuous exercise only gradually and with the advice and consent of your physician.* To avoid discomfort or infection, your feet should also be checked for unusual callus formation, which may point to faulty weight bearing. The condition of your heart and eyes should also be checked.

Food and Type II diabetes

Managing one's PEEP is an important link in the chain of events for the person with non-insulin-dependent diabetes. If you refer to the beginning of Chapter 8, you will see that your overall goals, if you are an overweight adult, are to reach and to maintain the weight that you and your physician decide is optimal for you and to maintain a good level of physical activity. It may seem hard to do this, but if it can be accomplished, the rewards are great. It is possible that the symptoms of diabetes (fatigue, frequent infections, increased thirst, and urination) can disappear and the blood sugar can return to normal. After the early period of adjustment, you will have more energy and less afternoon and evening drowsiness. Then you will feel more like exerting yourself.

You may have been given reducing diets before and found it difficult to lose weight. Or you may have achieved weight loss by means of "crash" diets or periods of starvation, but then promptly regained it all. As you know, the principle behind weight loss is, of course, to eat less food than you actually need for each day's activities. The best way to increase the gap between the calories you take in and the calories you expend is to increase your activity. In fact, once you have lost weight and reversed your diabetic state, this may be the only way that you can keep your weight down and stay feeling fit. This usually means that you will have to change some parts of your daily life-style, as described in the sections on day-to-day management and physical fitness in Chapter 8.

Many people find that at the beginning they lose weight easily and rapidly. However, further weight loss may be disappointingly slow. There are reasons for these slowing-down periods, called plateaus. Much of the successful loss in the beginning may be of body fluid rather than fat. Later, when real weight has been lost, the metabolic rate of the body actually drops. The body senses that fewer calories are available and slows down its machinery as a survival reaction. Therefore few calories are needed for weight loss to occur. It is at this point that deliberate increase in physical activity becomes particularly useful. These plateaus will sometimes occur despite careful adjustments in decreasing food intake and increasing physical activity. Plateaus can occur for two other reasons. First, the body will "hold on" to fluid when it senses that there is less bulk in one's food intake. The kidneys retain salt and water, which is eventually released as fluid as fat stores continue to drop. Secondly, as one's exercise program develops, muscle tissue will replace fat stores. Since muscle weighs more than fat, your weight may stabilize, despite dietary efforts and an increase in physical activity.

The purpose of all reducing diet plans for non-insulin-dependent diabetics is to burn up fat and minimize the demands for insulin. There are two reasons for minimizing the demand for insulin. First, you want to preserve your own insulin-producing capability for as long as you can. Second, insulin itself promotes the storage of excess food as fat. Therefore, the most important thing is for you to cut down on your total caloric intake. Ideally, weight reduction diets, like normal diets, should provide food selections that are nutritionally balanced. They should contain from 12% to 20% of calories as protein, 30% to 38% as fat, and 50% to 60% as carbohydrate, although the amount of food is strictly limited. The body needs all these forms of food for good health. Also, a pleasant variety of foods can be included even when the total number of calories is small. Of course, people vary in their energy needs according to the type of life they lead. Obviously, an overweight construction worker needs more calories than an overweight professor, even when reducing.

In addition to low-calorie, nutritionally-balanced meal plans, various forms of acutely restricted diets can be used under close medical supervision. At times, this approach is appropriate and can help you to break the vicious cycle of increasing weight and insulin resistance. You can look at this period of time as a "starting-over period, wiping the slate clean." Total starvation is, of course, the most drastic and rapid method of weight loss, but for every pound of fat lost, a third of a pound of valuable body protein is also lost. Therefore, instead of complete starvation, some protein is often provided with variable amounts of carbohydrate. This is called the protein-supplemented modified fast. The demand for insulin is minimized on this diet. These approaches to weight loss are still quite experimental and are being constantly modified. However, you and your physician may want to consider such a program as part of your overall plan to help you lose weight rapidly to a point where you can exercise more comfortably. These diets may be dangerous if not carefully supervised.

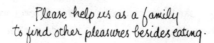

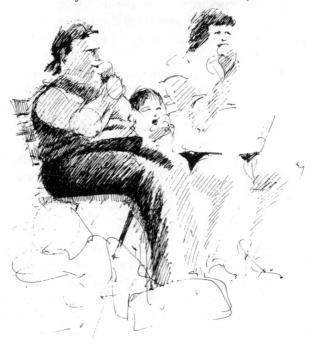

Before you start on a very restrictive program, or for that matter, any conscious change in eating habits, we encourage spending some time (5 to 7 days) tuning into eating habits. You can look at yourself as a personal scientist or newspaper reporter—getting the facts that will allow you better insight into your food selection and eating habits. One way to collect information is to keep records, and you can use your imagination in this process. Some individuals find using a monthly calendar helpful because they can clearly see each day and pinpoint trends. Other approaches are journals, which include food intake, records of physical activity and events, thoughts or feelings that have occurred each day. The use of tables and graphs, as outlined in *Eating Is Okay!* and *Permanent Weight Control* can also be helpful.*

Your diet counselor can also help you to manage your diabetes and avoid the necessity of taking insulin by taking a careful dietary and activi-

---

*See Appendix A for complete references.

ty history from you and then suggesting certain changes that will help to bring down your blood sugar level while losing and/or maintaining your ideal weight. Sample menus can be planned, taking into account your food likes and dislikes. After awhile, you will become knowledgeable about all kinds of food and very skilled at planning your own menues. You will develop new and wiser diet habits and feel better because of it. You will also save money on your food bills! One of the advantages of your kind of diabetes is that you don't have to watch the clock all the time. Missing or delaying a meal is not harmful to those who do not take insulin, as it may be to those who take insulin or oral medication. However, this doesn't mean that you make up for the delayed or missed meal by eating more at the next meal. Remember that your body cannot handle an excess of food. It is important to realize that if you are being treated with an oral medication, hypoglycemia (low blood sugar) can occur. This is especially so if there are changes in food intake such as skipping or delaying meals. If you are taking an oral medication, you should be aware of signs and symptoms of low blood sugar levels that are described in Chapter 10.

Chapter 10
Health maintenance

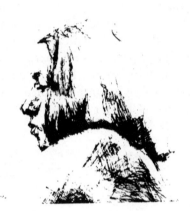

Do you know how I can get in touch with other diabetics?

Testing blood and urine for well days and sick days

The aim of monitoring blood and urine in Type II diabetes is to see whether you can keep your diabetes under control. You may *think you feel fine* because you are used to feeling less than well. But remember the goals set forth in Chapter 8 and all the reasons for protecting your pancreas, blood vessels, and nerves!

In Chapter 4, we described SBGM and urine testing and urged people with either type of diabetes to learn to use both types of tests. People with Type II diabetes do not need to test as often as Type I diabetics because they are not in danger of sudden insulin reactions. However, blood testing for non-insulin-dependent persons is a valuable resource for the following reasons:

1. Testing your own blood will show you dramatically what happens in your body when you eat, how that varies according to the kinds and amounts of food, and what effect exercise has on the blood glucose. Blood testing teaches and rewards you and can be a source of encouragement to persevere.
2. In people who have had diabetes for many years, sometimes without knowing it, the kidney may develop an increased ability to retain glucose in the blood above 180. It is therefore quite possible to have a high blood sugar level without sugar appearing in the urine as a warning. If you know how to test your blood, you can check your kidney function. Test the blood and a second-voided urine at the same time and compare the results. Then you know whether or not you can rely on urine testing some of the time.
3. If you are sick, it is a great comfort to you and your doctor to know what your blood glucose is from hour to hour.

When to test

In the beginning, blood and urine testing will tell you whether you are successfully reducing the resistance to your own insulin. During this period, test at least several times a week and pick the times when you are most likely to have a high blood sugar, such as 1 to 2 hours after your largest meal. If you are spilling glucose at that time, test again before breakfast. If either of these tests is positive for glucose on a regular basis, consult your doctor or nurse to see whether changes in your daily plan should be considered. Keep a record of what you have eaten and your schedule of exercise as well as the time and result of the test.

After you have stabilized at a good weight and learned your pattern of response to food and exercise, the purpose of testing is to keep track of any changes in your body. If things are going smoothly, a blood or urine check twice a week may often be enough.

Sick day guidelines

If you are ill, test several times a day for blood glucose and ketones. In the event of a bad cold, gastrointestinal upset, injury, or unusual stress, test daily or more often.

If you have consistently large amounts of sugar in the urine, call your doctor. If there is both sugar and more than a trace of acetone, notify your doctor without delay. Mild diabetes may become severe under the stress of illness. Infections with staphylococci, such as boils, are particularly prone to cause this reaction.

If you are borderline diabetic in the older age group, a condition known as *hyperosmolar coma* may develop when you are ill. This requires prompt, usually short-term treatment with insulin and fluids. In this case the blood sugar level rises very markedly, but ketones do not appear in the urine. A test that is strongly positive for glucose with progressive drowsiness is a sign you should call for help.

If you are unable to eat or are vomiting, you should seek help. A strongly positive test for acetone without glucose in the urine is a normal reaction to starvation, and glucose plus acetone may signify trouble. During acute illness, try to take sugar- or salt-containing fluids such as skimmed milk, ginger ale, or broth. However, if you are vomiting, do not keep taking fluids since they may increase vomiting, which in turn leads to dehydration.

If, for any special reason, you are taking oral agents for treatment of your diabetes and you are unable to eat, there is danger of serious and prolonged lowering of the blood sugar level. This applies particularly to the longer-acting drugs, such as Diabinase. Try to take some sugar-containing fluid regularly and *call your doctor*.

Pregnancy in Type II diabetes

The goal in pregnancy for Type II diabetes is the same as in Type I—to have a normal, healthy baby. This goal is realistic with modern methods (see Chapter 5). It is just as important to manage the diabetes carefully, but the daily self-care objectives of the two types of diabetes differ to some degree.

In non-insulin-dependent diabetes, the mother is still producing insulin. However, she has a tendency toward obesity and a resistance to insulin. If this tendency is allowed to get out of hand during the normal weight gain of pregnancy, it will be more difficult to keep the blood glucose within normal range because her resistance to insulin will increase. Therefore it is important to avoid gaining any more weight than absolutely necessary for the healthy development of the baby. Calories in a balanced diet should be limited to allow not much more than a weight gain of 15 pounds. The diet should take advantage of high fiber and a relatively high content of complex carbohydrates to limit wide swings in the blood glucose level. The mother must not fast since the ketones of even brief fasting may do harm to the baby. Moderate, regular exercise will help to maintain weight at the right level. If the blood glucose level cannot be kept within normal range by this method, insulin can be given. But it is still necessary to continue the diet and exercise program.

If you have Type II diabetes and are planning a pregnancy, consider going into training for it just the way an athlete does before a major competitive event. Physical fitness and good nutritional habits will be an asset to you and your child for many years to come. If you can keep your weight under control during pregnancy, your child may be less likely to develop obesity later in life. Your own diabetes will be more manageable, and your overall health will be better for years to come.

Foot care for those who have had diabetes for many years

The abnormal blood glucose level of diabetes over the years may gradually damage the nerves and blood vessels that carry messages and nourishment to the feet. Then they become numb, less sensitive to pain or discomfort, and more difficult to heal. It is possible to have a bruise, cut, or other injury, or even an infection and not notice that anything is wrong. Therefore the first rule in foot care is for you and your doctor to be aware of them.

1. Look at your feet every day!
2. Wash your feet daily with soap and warm water. Dry thoroughly, especially between the toes, patting rather than rubbing.
3. Rub with an emollient or moisturizer as needed to keep skin soft and free from scales and dryness. (Emollients are lanolin, mineral or vegetable oils, and Vaseline.) If you tend to get calluses, you may need to do this 2 to 3 times a week. Emery boards may be used carefully to smooth roughened areas before washing. Lamb's wool is a good material to protect sore places.
4. Use these times to examine your feet carefully for calluses, which may indicate faulty weight bearing. Our feet have evolved to carry most of the weight on the strong column of bones above the big toes. Sometimes, however, these bones are short and the weight is thrown on the second bone of the ball of the foot. In time, this may lead to the development of a callus, a good deal of discomfort, and even an ulcer. The thickness of your calluses shows how you are bearing weight. Look at them carefully. If you have an unequal build-up, consult your doctor. A simple innersole with a pad to throw the weight under the big toe again

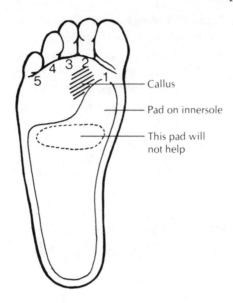

can avoid major problems. An arch-supporting pad under the entire ball of the foot will not help. When the heel is raised during walking, the weight will still be thrown on the second bone of the ball of the foot.

5. If you find that you have a rash, fungus, athlete's foot, or warts, consult your doctor. (A rash might be caused by allergies, psoriasis, eczema, or overuse of a remedy.) Don't use chemicals without consulting your doctor.

6. If the nails are brittle and dry, soften them by soaking them in warm water 10 to 15 minutes before cutting them. Clean gently around the nails with a soft brush and orangewood stick. Avoid probing with metal tools. Cut your nails in a good light, straight across and not too short. If you go to a podiatrist (foot doctor), tell him you have diabetes.

7. Socks or hose should be clean, absorbent, and fit comfortably to avoid pressure on the toenails. Articles of clothing such as narrow, tight, elastic garters or hose and sock tops can hinder circulation in the long blood vessels of the leg. Crossing the leg at the knee has the same effect. Try to avoid these hazards.

8. To avoid blisters and calluses, be sure to buy shoes of soft leather and good fit. Break in new shoes carefully, a little at a time. If you have poor sensation in your feet, avoid open-heeled and open-

toed shoes. If your feet vary in size because of swelling at the end of the day, it is a good idea to have one pair of shoes a size larger than usual.

9. When you go outside, wear shoes suitable for whatever activity is planned. Slippers do not provide enough protection outdoors. Do not go barefoot where you cannot see what is underfoot. Exercising toes in clean sand when swimming is beneficial, however.

10. Consult your doctor about any pain, redness, swelling, or any inflammation. If you develop pain in the *calves* of your legs *during* exercise, tell your doctor. This may mean that your circulation is not adequate.

11. When you get into the tub, test the water with your wrist before putting your feet in, especially if you have diminished sensation as you get older. Check regularly for areas of numbness.

12. Bedsocks are the safest way to keep feet warm in bed.

13. Remember that tobacco in any form decreases circulation to the feet.

14. If you have very poor circulation, arrange to sit with your feet up 5 or more minutes every hour of the day.

15. Perspiration of the feet can be a real hazard, not just a joking matter. It can be relieved by swabbing the feet with witch hazel and dusting lightly with antiseptic powder. Sole inserts available with activated charcoal cut down on odor caused by bacteria, but the shoe needs to be large enough to accommodate them. Plastic shoes combined with nylon hose increase perspiration. Cotton footwear absorbs moisture best. Canvas or leather shoes are much better than artificial materials or rubber.

16. Exercise the feet and legs daily to increase circulation because the massaging action of the leg muscles improves circulation.
    a. Bend each foot down and up as far as it will go 6 times.
    b. Make a circle to the left, then to the right, 6 times.
    c. Raise on tiptoes 6 to 12 times.
    d. *Walk regularly!*

The oral agents

Many adult Type II diabetics take pills to bring down their blood glucose level. These pills are called oral or hypoglycemic agents, to distinguish them from insulin. Insulin cannot be given by mouth since it is digested like any other protein and is not absorbed through the intestinal tract. Oral agents work in an entirely different way. Brand names of the oral agents in use today include Orinase, Tolinase, Diabinese, Dymelor, Glyburide, and Glucotrol (Glipizide).

In recent years, there has been a lot of debate about the effectiveness, side effects, and danger of the oral agents. Many physicians and people with Type II diabetes are not certain about using them. The biggest problem with oral agents in the 1960s and 1970s was that we thought of them as a "cure." Since it is such a difficult task to lose weight, everyone was happy to think that people could take medication and stop worrying. At that time, not very much was known about the many mechanisms underlying this type of diabetes and the fact that these mechanisms vary a great deal from person to person. No one realized then how much being overweight and inactive contributes to resistance to insulin.

But now that development of oral agents is going through a phase of expansion and research, there is a new "second generation" of medications that may be more effective in smaller doses. In addition, there is greater understanding of the different ways in which each oral agent may act to overcome the various defects that cause non-insulin-dependent diabetes. When we have good methods of pinpointing the exact defects, it will be easier for doctors to choose the best medication for each individual.

Oral agents make two very valuable contributions for some people. First, they help to correct the inherited slower-than-normal release of insulin after meals. Second, they directly or indirectly lower resistance to insulin. Serum insulin goes down, and the number of receptors on the cells goes up again. Recent research suggests that the oral agents may also improve the body's use of glucose in the large muscles.

There are some disadvantages to oral agents, aside from costs. First, these medications are not effective if they are taken as a substitute for diet and exercise. Persons with Type II diabetes who take oral agents may think that things are going well if they do not have to get up in the night any more. However, there may still be high blood glucose levels that will not be discovered by urine tests alone (see Chapter 4). In the meantime, blood vessels and nerves may be slowly damaged, leading to those all-too-familiar complications with vision, sexuality, kidneys, and heart. Second, there is a high percentage of people for whom the oral agents do not work for very long. So far, less than one half of those using oral agents remain in control of their diabetes for more than 3 years.

If you are taking oral agents now or if you and your physician are thinking of using them, you may wish to consider the following points:

1. Remember that SBGM will tell you whether or not your treatment plan is working and guide you as you make changes.

2. Remember that oral agents will not work without your PEEP.
3. Be sure that you and your physician carefully choose the right oral agent for you and that you take the right dose, working up to it gradually.
4. If you have lost your extra weight and increased your activity level, you and your physician may want to schedule a well-supervised trial period without the pills. There is no sense in taking medicine if you can do without it.

Stay in touch with the American Diabetes Association in regard to the new developments. Read *Diabetes Forecast* magazine. Prevail in your life-long rehabilitation!

Part III
Insulin-dependent Type I diabetes

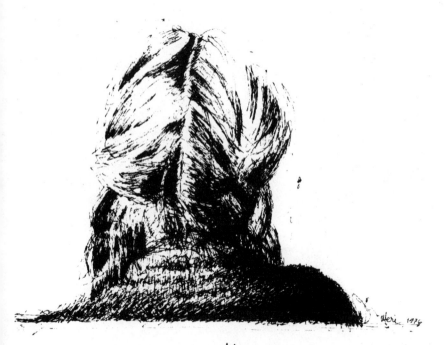

Help me count my strengths —
Remind me that I'm going to feel well again.

Chapter 11
Goals for insulin-dependent Type I persons

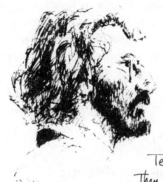

Teach me the trade-offs.
Then let me choose my routines.

Learn how your body works

1. To grow and develop normally.
2. To be active in work and recreation.
3. To preserve healthy blood vessels and nerves to all parts of your body by keeping your blood glucose as near normal as possible. This will help to protect your heart, your brain, your sexuality, your eyesight, your kidneys.

Plan

1. There is more than one method and schedule by which you can live with diabetes. Learn what your options are. Consider how to take your food and insulin in a manner as close as possible to the way the normal body functions. Be willing to try different ways

of doing things. Learn the new techniques for testing your own blood and for giving insulin.

2. When you eat and when you exercise, think about these events in relation to each other and to your insulin dose.

3. Learn how to use sugars in many forms in combination with other foods to help you to keep going during exercise, to protect you against low blood sugar levels, to make up for unplanned physical activity or changes in your schedule.

4. Check your supplies of insulin, syringes, testing materials, and emergency food packets every day. Bring them with you all the time so that you will be protected as you go about your regular life activities. If you are ever out of control, it need not be for long if you have the tools at hand to bring back your balance. Look at your diet sheet for suggestions of foods to carry.

5. Keep in regular touch with your health care team. Your needs will change as you grow. You need to stay up-to-date on new information about diabetes. For example, you will want to hear how the insulin pump is developing. Join your local or national diabetes association and read *Diabetes Forecast* magazine.

6. Get a medical identification emblem and wear it at all times.

Insulin action in the body
Insulin response to food, normal and diabetic

You have many choices open to you for the management of your diabetes. You and your physician should explore them together to find out what will work best for you. The old idea that there was one right way to take insulin has been discarded. There are many right ways, and you can try them out without a sense of failure if the daily plan needs to be changed. It is now recognized that individuals vary, one from another, a great deal in their response to insulin. Furthermore, each individual will vary somewhat from day to day as a result of variations in activity, level of stress, food intake, and the rate at which insulin is absorbed, depending on where it was injected. Some people even have a different insulin schedule for weekends or vacations than the one they use during a regular work schedule. In this section, we will look at what insulin does in the body, types of insulin available today, and some examples of insulin schedules.

Fig. 6 shows how the nondiabetic pancreas responds to food to keep the blood glucose level within the normal range. Insulin is secreted right at the time of meals, and glucose never rises above 160 mg/dl.

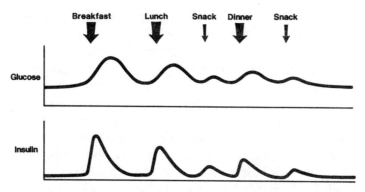

fig. 6 Normal pattern of glucose rise and fall as it is controlled by insulin release.

You can see that the variations in the blood glucose level are quite small. This control is accomplished in two ways. First, a small but very important amount of insulin is secreted continuously, providing an essential background. Until recently it was thought that this background insulin was all that mattered. However, early in the 1970s it was found that, at the time of meals, even before the blood glucose has begun to rise, insulin is secreted into the bloodstream quite rapidly. The sight of a meal alone triggers the secretion of insulin, even before eating. We now know that this insulin is the most significant in controlling blood glucose. Your goal is to take insulin to come as close as possible to this normal pattern.

Insulin has three functions in the body. First, when we eat, insulin brings the carbohydrates in food into body cells for immediate energy. Second, it helps to store fuels for later use in two forms—glycogen in the liver and muscle cells and fat in the fat deposits. Third, insulin helps to move amino acids, the building blocks of protein, into cells.

To keep the body nourished during changes in activity, another group of hormones is important as messengers in the body's information system. They are called the counterregulatory hormones because they balance the blood sugar–lowering actions of insulin. Some of these hormones come from the pancreas, such as glucagon and somatostatin. Others come from the adrenal glands, such as cortisol and epinephrine. They respond to a low blood sugar level by increasing resistance to insulin and by breaking down the glycogen stored in the liver to release glucose for energy. Glucagon also helps to make glucose from protein.

It is not possible with the methods we have today to mimic the automatic way in which these hormones work together in the normal body. In addition, injecting insulin one or more times a day into an arm, the abdomen, or a leg does not give the same effect as having the blood pick it up from the pancreas. The timing in relation to meals and exercise is not as precise, and the insulin is not delivered into the blood through the portal vein. This vein drains directly into the liver, the chemical factory in the body where reserves of energy are stored. Research in developing an artificial pancreas and the present availability of open-loop insulin pumps are big steps in the right direction (see Chapter 12). In the meantime, people who have insulin-dependent diabetes have to do a lot of thinking for the pancreas to avoid extreme variations in blood glucose. Even with everyone's best efforts, there will be times when the blood glucose level will be too high or too low. It is important to be realistic about what can be achieved so as not to feel angry or guilty when it is not necessary. But it is even more important to strike the best bargain you can with your diabetes, both for daily wellness and for long-term health.

Stages of insulin-dependent diabetes

Type I diabetes develops in stages. Everyone used to think that when insulin-dependent diabetes first developed, it was always a sudden event that made the person very sick. However, recently, it has been discovered that Type I diabetes may be developing for quite a long time before it comes into the open. Researchers have been studying family members known to be at risk of Type I diabetes, such as the twin of a person with diabetes. They find that an individual may have antibodies to insulin in the blood for several years without symptoms. These antibodies are evidence of the autoimmune reaction discussed in Chapter 1. This surprising fact has created interest in trying to suppress the autoimmune response and thus preserve the pancreas.

During this very early stage, the release of insulin may be delayed and also abnormally prolonged, producing a low blood sugar level 4 to 5 hours after a meal, along with the symptoms typical of an insulin reaction. Afternoon irritability and confusion may be an early warning sign of insulin-dependent diabetes.

When a person actually develops diabetes, there is an acute need for insulin at first. But then he or she may have a "honeymoon period" lasting weeks or even months when no injected insulin is required. This is the result of a temporary recovery in the ability to secrete insulin. Researchers are now studying this period to see if diabetes could be reversed or postponed. Techniques are now available to reduce the autoimmune response. Unfortunately, they also lower the body's entire defense system against illness. Much work remains to be done before we can count on reversing Type I diabetes in the first phase. During the second phase of diabetes, some insulin may be secreted before meals, but later on, the ability to produce any insulin is completely lost. At this point, two or more injections of insulin a day are necessary to keep the body healthy.

Insulin preparations for the 1980s

There are many types of insulin on the market today. They vary in degree of purity, how closely they match the human insulin molecule, length of action in the body, and in cost. Let's begin by looking at the different sources of insulin preparations.

Insulin has been made from beef or pork pancreas for many years. Pork insulin is closest to human insulin in the structure of its molecule. Most commercial insulin is a combination of 90% beef and 10% pork. Pure beef or pure pork insulin costs twice as much. Human insulin has recently been made available by using bacteria to make parts of the insulin molecule, which are then joined together by very sophisticated laboratory methods. Various synthetic insulins are now on the market at considerable cost. These costs may come down gradually with competition.

Several companies now offer a variety of insulins. Lilly and Squibb are well-known American companies. Squibb has combined with a Danish company and is now called Squibb-Novo. Another Danish company is Nordisk. They all make good insulins. Shop around for what's best for you.

People ask, why buy expensive insulin? If the customary beef-pork insulin is working well for you, there may be no need to shift. However, especially for a person who has just recently developed diabetes, there is some evidence that the purer insulins closest to human insulin may reduce the antibodies that build up to insulin taken over the life span. In addition, some people develop allergies to insulin, and the purest products reduce this problem.

Types of insulins

In addition to the choice of preparation of insulin, there are two main classes of insulin available, in terms of the length of time they take to act in the body.

Short-acting, "regular" or "clear" insulin

These are zinc salts of unmodified insulin, are absorbed relatively rapidly, and have the shortest duration of action.

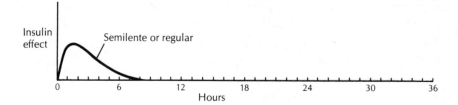

Modified insulin

In modified insulin, the absorption is slowed and the action is prolonged by either combining with another protein or by modifying the crystalline structure. The four most common American preparations are: (1) *semilente insulin,* which acts in much the same way as "regular" insulin; (2) *NPH insulin,* which consists of a stable mixture of two parts of regular short-acting insulin to one part of neutral protamine longer-acting insulin; (3) *lente insulin,* which has essentially the same pattern of action as NPH; and (4) *ultralente,* which is extremely long-acting. All modified insulins are cloudy in appearance. Squibb-Novo and Nordisk insulins of excellent quality are now widely available in all the same classes—short-acting, intermediate, and long-acting—and in various combinations of beef, pork, and synthetic human insulin. Ask your physician about them—they may work for you.

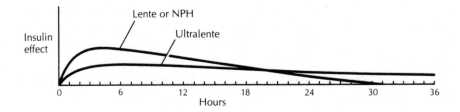

Onset, peak, and duration of action of insulins

From the preceding diagrams you can see that the time at which insulin begins to take effect is somewhat the same. Insulin has to combine with body cells as it is absorbed from under the skin, which takes 20 to 30 minutes. Therefore the injection should be given well before eating.

Table 5. Variations between individual responses to insulin

Type	Onset (hr)	Peak (hr)	Duration (hr)
Regular or semilente	½–1	2–8	5–12
NPH or lente	½–1	6–12	24–28
Ultralente	Gradual	18–24	36+

CAUTION: The time of action of all insulins varies from person to person.

As far as the peak action and the length of action of the different preparations, there is a *wide range and a lot of variation between individuals in their response to insulin*. Table 5 demonstrates these variations.

As with everything else in diabetes, only trial and error and trial again will teach you how your body responds to insulin. Just to make things even more complicated, insulin action may also vary within one person. This will depend in part on the site of injection and the nature of the body tissues. Insulin is absorbed rapidly from muscle and most evenly from just under the skin. It will be absorbed slowly from fatty areas of the body such as the buttocks. It is absorbed most efficiently from the abdomen, next most efficiently from the arms, and least efficiently from the thighs. You can learn to take these variations into consideration in choosing your injection site, along with thinking about your blood glucose level at the time and your plans for the next few hours. Keeping a record for your own use is a great help, especially in the beginning. Then you can see at a glance what your pattern of response is to food, exercise, and insulin for a week at a time. You can design a record sheet of your own or ask your American Diabetes Association affiliate to recommend a source. The *Diabetic's 365-Day Medical Diary* (St. Louis, 1983, The C.V. Mosby Co.) is a good example.

Chapter 12
Day-to-day management of insulin-dependent diabetes: you have options

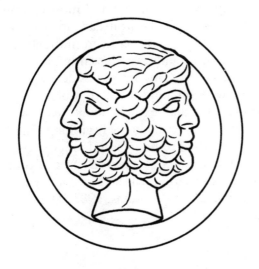

Like the Roman god Janus who guarded doors and gates, you need to look both ways to keep the fuel in your body in the right traffic lanes.

This chapter will provide a few examples of the many possible insulin schedules and a discussion of the insulin pump so you will have an idea of the range of options open to you. But, before we begin, take another look at the diagram in Chapter 11, which shows the normal pattern of rise and fall of glucose in the nondiabetic person. Remember that the goal is to come as close to that as possible. Then review Chapter 4 on monitoring diabetes with blood and urine tests. SBGM is almost as important to you as insulin itself.

Your blood tests will help in two ways. First, you know what your blood glucose is before you eat and that helps in looking ahead to decide how much insulin to take, when to take it, and whether or not to exercise. Second, if your blood glucose is not in the normal range, it helps you to look backward to find out why so you can avoid the problem the next day.

Insulin injection schedules

It is nearly impossible to control blood glucose rise after meals with a single morning injection without having insulin reactions at other times of the day. Therefore many physicians today agree that the best way to begin is to take two injections (split dose) of intermediate-acting insulin such as NPH or lente, one before breakfast and the other before the evening meal (Fig. 7). The following diagram shows how insulin takes effect on this schedule. Sensitivity to insulin increases during the day, and no major meals are eaten at night. Therefore the evening dose can usually be about half the morning dose. The blood test before breakfast will guide you to decide the minimum amount of evening insulin that will maintain a normal blood glucose overnight. The test before the evening meal will tell you whether you took enough insulin that morning to last through the rest of the day without an insulin reaction.

Many people who want to lead lives that call for lots of flexibility and the ability to move fast have decided that 3 or 4 injections of insulin each day are worth the effort. Not only do these people feel energetic for more hours of the day when the blood glucose is within the normal range, but they are free of the rigid meal schedule. Best of all, they know that they are providing themselves with the best long-term health insurance they

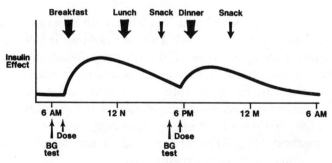

fig. 7 Split dose of intermediate-acting insulin.

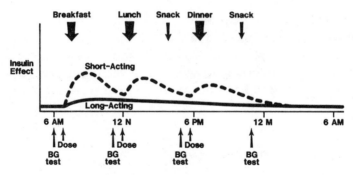

fig. 8 Short-acting insulin before each meal with long-acting insulin added to the morning injection.

have because this plan comes closest to the way the normal body functions. Another advantage is that if their blood glucose level does get out of control, it is only 3 to 4 hours until their next insulin injection. Their blood glucose level will never be high for many hours at a stretch, and it is the overall average for the day that counts.

Combining insulins with different action periods can go a long way toward mimicking the normal pancreas. Remember the trickle of background insulin in the nondiabetic pancreas? Fig. 8 is a diagram of an insulin schedule that is often used today. A small amount of ultralente is used in the breakfast dose along with regular insulin, and regular insulin is used before each of the other meals throughout the day. Some people need a small amount of insulin with the bedtime snack. Others do not. Some people can get along without the ultralente, just using 3 or 4 injections of regular insulin.

Table 6 provides examples of different insulin schedules. The great thing about combining these options with SBGM is that you eventually realize that you can think for your pancreas and make adjustments in your daily care as necessary. There may be other combinations that work for you.

At this point you may say that it looks like a lot of work. You may ask, "Are there simpler options?" What about nasal insulin? What about the insulin pumps? In regard to nasal insulin, the only advantage is that you don't have to use a needle. In time, it may become a reliable option, but at present, there are many variables to contend with as far as rate of absorption is concerned. It is purely experimental at this point. In addition, you still have to do all the thinking, adjusting, and testing required by the other methods. Insulin pumps really are a new departure and are described and evaluated in the following pages.

Table 6. Different insulin schedules

Breakfast	Lunch	Supper	Bedtime	Comments
NPH or lente		NPH or lente		A good beginning
Ultralente and regular	Regular	Regular		Mimics normal
Regular	Regular	Regular		Works for people in whom regular insulin has long action
NPH and regular		Regular	NPH	No noon injection
Regular	Regular	Regular and NPH		No bedtime injection
Regular	Regular	Regular	NPH	No mixtures

Insulin pumps

The recent electronic and technological revolution has brought with it the dream of an artificial pancreas: a device that would replace the damaged, insulin-producing beta cells and effortlessly produce perfect blood sugar control. People with diabetes would then be able to dispense with the shots, the finger-sticks, the urine tests, and the myriad of decisions and discomforts they encounter day after day.

For many years, scientists were convinced that an artificial pancreas must be able to measure blood sugar concentrations. How else would it be able to calculate the proper dose of insulin? This information would be fed to a tiny computer that would control a small pump that was connected to a reservoir of stored insulin. Finally, just the right amount of insulin would be delivered at the right times to the space surrounding the intestines (peritoneum) or directly into the blood vessels feeding the liver.

Some parts of the artificial pancreas are relatively easy to make. For example, the computer directing the flow of insulin is quite manageable. On the other hand, the continuous and reliable measurement of the blood sugar level in the body is a particularly difficult task. Nevertheless, the combined efforts of engineers and physicians have produced a relatively primitive, artificial pancreas. It is large (suitcase sized), impractical, finicky, very expensive, and obviously much too big to be carried around. Since they will operate for only a few days (with constant, expert technical attention), these machines are only practical for scientific research.

Sometimes, though, bigger and more complex isn't necessarily better. It came as somewhat of a surprise that mechanical insulin-delivery systems may not need to directly measure the blood sugar level. A relatively simple machine, an insulin pump, that does little more than give insulin at a steady rate (basal rate) between meals and a little extra before meals (bolus) can do a good job. When it is used with home blood glucose monitoring by someone who is self-reliant, has a little mechanical ability, and has a good attitude about his or her insulin-dependent diabetes, the resulting blood sugar values can be quite close to normal nearly all the time. However, the person using the pump still has to be the thinking link, using personal measurements of blood glucose levels to determine the amounts of insulin to be injected by the pump. The user must accurately and frequently perform blood sugar tests and think ahead about meals and exercise before setting the controls on the device that regulate the rates of insulin delivery.

These pumps are small, battery powered, and all variations on the same theme. They inject insulin through a thin tube leading to a small needle (a normal, 27-gauge insulin needle) taped into the skin of the belly. Some pumps simply use a motor to slowly push the plunger of an insulin-filled syringe, while others use roller pumps that squeeze the insulin through the tubing. They are easily hooked to the belt, worn in a special pouch, or just put into a shirt pocket. The available devices vary in size from about that of a deck of playing cards to a small paperback novel. They are worn 24 hours a day and only briefly removed to bathe or, every few days, to change the needle and tubing.

The first scientific reports of this type of therapy were exciting. Here, at last, was a treatment that could produce normal blood sugar concentrations for long periods. There were reports of reversal of eye disease and a decrease in the amount of protein lost to the urine from kidneys injured by diabetes. Could it be that these complications are reversible or, at least, preventable?

However, as more people used the pumps, several minor and serious problems came to light. There were infections under the skin where the needle had been left in place. Batteries wore out, needles came loose, pumps failed, and people made mistakes, all of which resulted in both ketoacidosis and low blood sugar episodes. It was clear that the same day-to-day problems of diabetes were shared by people who gave themselves their insulin by conventional injection and by people who used the insulin pump. There was even some concern that diabetic complications might happen more frequently and be more serious to pump-users. Several deaths, apparently related to hypoglycemia, prompted the Centers for Disease Control to investigate whether pump-users were, indeed, at increased risk for very serious complications. After all, unless someone shuts it off, the pump keeps giving insulin even during a low blood sugar episode. Fortunately, to the great relief of many people, this study found that the use of pumps was not associated with any unusual risks. In fact, there was a tendency for pump-users to have slightly fewer problems than the total diabetic population.

All the facts about insulin pumps are not yet available. Meanwhile, though, everyone with Type I diabetes, in consultation with his or her doctor, has some difficult decisions to make. The use of an insulin pump may be an appropriate choice for some people, but how does one decide if the pump will fit into one's personal treatment plan?

1. *Consider the cost of insulin pump therapy.* The purchase price of the pump ranges from $1000 to $3000. A hospital stay of 3 to 7 days is often required to supervise the initial stages of treatment and to familiarize the person with diabetes with this new way of administering insulin. Supplies (for home blood glucose monitoring, needles, tubing, syringes, and the like) may cost $10 to $20 per week. Some insurance plans cover some or all of these expenses. At the present time the cost per year is approximately $1000.

2. *Consider the commitment.* Safe and successful pump therapy is clearly related to the motivation and willingness of the user to adhere to an intensive and rigid schedule of home blood glucose monitoring. The pump-user must be able to make wise, often independent decisions regarding the daily insulin doses. The pump is best used by someone who accepts these responsibilities and realizes that the pump is not, unfortunately, a "cure." The pump, after all, is nothing more than a convenient way of administering insulin. Some people find it a lot easier than the other methods that can produce equally good results such as multiple, daily shots of insulin. It is also possible and sometimes necessary to go back and forth between pumps and multiple, daily shots depending on one's particular activity.

3. *Consider the available resources.* Doctors who are experienced with pump therapy know that the teaching and supervision of patients using insulin pumps demands special skills and lots of time. Make sure your doctor is trained to do this. A well-organized teaching program should be provided for persons beginning pump therapy. Also ask whether or not skilled, professional coverage is available on a 24-hour basis.

4. *Consider the fact that the pump is often worn outside your clothes, and it*

may tell people that you have diabetes. Are you comfortable talking to others about your diabetes? People will, undoubtedly, casually ask you about that "thing" hanging from your belt.

5. *Consider the alternatives to pump therapy* if you're just striving for good control of your diabetes. Most studies have shown comparable results between the average blood sugar achieved with pump therapy and intensive, flexible, conventional management by 3 to 5 injections a day. However, it is not yet known whether people with certain types of diabetes will actually do better with one form of therapy or another. Many people, however, are devoted fans of insulin pump therapy simply for the convenience it offers and the good results they've experienced with it. Remember, having good, steady blood sugar has its own rewards, regardless of how you accomplish it.

6. *Consider carefully your choice of a pump.* Many companies are now making pumps and marketing them aggressively. As a result of a quirk in the law governing medical devices, pumps do not have to undergo any patient testing before they are sold. It is wise, therefore, to select a model that has been around a while. Furthermore, don't spend more money than necessary. Some pumps are equipped with expensive features such as clocks and the ability to change rates automatically several times a day. It is not yet clear whether these features are really necessary. All pumps are also subject to mechanical failure. Good support from the manufacturer is a necessity.

7. *Consider the advice of someone who is using or has used a pump.* Nothing can be more valuable than a frank discussion with someone who is using an insulin pump. Your doctor might be able to give you the name of someone willing to help you decide. You should try to find out the plusses and minuses before you make the commitment.

8. *Consider the situations in which use of the pump would be especially beneficial or harmful.* Some doctors believe that the pump is a blessing to the pregnant, Type I diabetic woman, while others strongly disagree. There is, however, no argument over the fact that tight control during the entire pregnancy has great rewards for mother and child. It probably doesn't matter very much how good control is achieved. On the other hand, sometimes the pump just isn't the right solution. For example, experience has told us that the person who is suffering from repeated episodes of ketoacidosis and hypoglycemia will, most likely, have the same problems using a pump. Overweight, Type II diabetic people are also inappropriate candidates for pump therapy. They should focus their efforts on weight loss and exercise.

In summary, it is clear that the insulin pump is not a "cure" for diabetes and it is not the "artificial pancreas." It is a compromise. In exchange for simplicity and size, the safe and successful use of the pump demands that the user willingly and unfailingly accept the burdens and responsibilities of insulin-dependent diabetes, day after day. Unfortunately, those who most need good diabetes control are sometimes the least likely to accept the many daily chores imposed by the pump or, for that matter, any form of intensive therapy. Instead of a pump, such persons need lots of patience and will have to wait for the day that the artificial pancreas or pancreatic transplant is a reality.

Chapter 13
Insulin treatment: cautions and skills

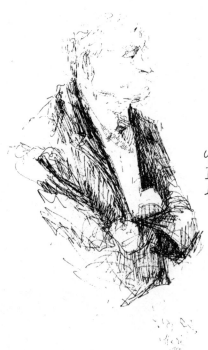

Young man,
you may be a doctor, but
I've had diabetes since
before you were born!

Trying to correct blood glucose by changing the wrong insulin dose

If you run a high blood sugar level at the same time of day for several days, do not take more insulin at the next dose to correct it. First, consider whether you may have a temporary cause such as an infection. Next, look at your record to see how much insulin you took *before* the high blood sugar level. Then plan to increase that dose the next day. For example, if you are taking two injections a day and if you have a high blood sugar level at 4 PM, you need to increase your next *morning* dose. Do not add to your 6 PM dose. The same process would apply to a low blood sugar level, except that you would *reduce* the dose. This process applies to people who use pumps as well as needles.

Making diabetes more severe with too much insulin: the Dawn Phenomenon and the Somogyi reaction

The Dawn phenomenon and the Somogyi reaction are two quite common events that can lead to trouble if we do not recognize them for what they are and distinguish between them.

Most people with Type I diabetes do not need more than 20 to 40 units of insulin a day. Some people take more insulin than they need and have insulin reactions without recognizing them. If a person with diabetes has a prolonged reaction to too much insulin, the body behaves as if it were starved. It draws on its stores of glycogen in the liver to raise blood glucose. When this reserved glycogen is used up, the body then shifts to burning fats, and ketones spill into the urine (see Chapter 4). In other words, what may have been mild diabetes will be made temporarily worse by too much insulin. If the insulin reaction is gradual and without acute symptoms, it is quite possible not to realize that it has happened at all, especially at night during sleep. If you then increase your insulin in response to a high blood glucose and possibly ketones in the urine, you will just make matters worse. The same thing will happen all over again, and you will appear to be a "brittle diabetic," hypersensitive and resistant to insulin all at the same time. This situation is called the Somogyi reaction. Your difficulties may disappear if you gradually lower your insulin dosage.

Another cause for high blood glucose levels in the morning is called

the Dawn phenomenon. In some people, whether or not they have diabetes, the blood glucose rises naturally between 4 AM and 6 AM. Some
people with diabetes may also exhibit this trait, and they may or may not
need extra evening insulin to compensate for it. In making that decision,
it is important to realize that it is the average 24-hour blood glucose that
counts. This is where the HgA1c test will help because it is important not
to take extra insulin and then have prolonged nighttime insulin reactions. The best way to find out whether a high blood glucose level in the
morning is a result of the Dawn phenomenon or a Somogyi reaction is to
set your alarm clock for 2 AM and do a blood test. If your blood glucose
level is below 60, you obviously do not need more insulin; you need less
at your evening dose or more to eat for your bedtime snack.

The following signs may indicate that you are taking too much insulin:
1. An apparent need for more than 50 units of insulin a day.
2. A urine test in the morning showing no glucose but positive for
   ketones.
3. A low morning temperature. The body temperature drops for a
   period of 6 hours or more after an insulin reaction. A check of
   morning temperature may be useful in finding out if you have reactions in the night.
4. Morning headache, perspiring during the night; restlessness, bad
   dreams, or apprehension at night.

If you have any of these symptoms, do not take additional insulin. You
and your physician should consider whether to lower or redistribute
your insulin doses, particularly those doses relating to the times of insulin reactions. If you are spilling ketones, you might need extra insulin
temporarily to restore control, but the long-term aim should be to reduce the amount of insulin. "Brittle" diabetics taking as much as 70 to
100 units of insulin a day can often reduce this to 30 to 40 units, readjust
the meal plan, and exercise and achieve steady control.

Effects of unstable diabetes on emotions

A person experiencing marked swings from high to low levels of
blood sugar will not feel well and may be irritable, depressed, tired, or
appear uncooperative. Such responses are quite often misinterpreted by
family, friends, or physician, and the person is accused of deliberately not
cooperating in the management of the diabetes. When a young person is
involved, this situation can lead to a lot of family misery, misunderstand-

ing, and needless conflict. If the blood sugar swings can be leveled out, these problems may disappear.

Delay in emptying the stomach as a cause of nighttime hypoglycemia

Another source of difficulty in achieving steady control may be delayed gastric emptying. This is not a common problem, and it usually only occurs after having diabetes for many years, but it is important to recognize it. It is one of the neuropathies caused by a disturbance of the nerves that control the movement of the internal organs. Signs that this problem exists are weight loss, lack of appetite, and a sense of fullness before the end of a meal. Sometimes there may be regurgitation of stomach contents many hours after eating. Difficulty in swallowing or bouts of diarrhea at night may also occur.

This slow emptying of the stomach causes a delay in digestion so that the body does not get the full nutritional value of the meal at the usual time. A result, therefore, may be an unexpected low blood sugar level, especially at night, with an exaggeration of the Somogyi reaction. An x-ray study of the upper gastrointestinal tract can establish the diagnosis. Simple measures, such as reducing the amount of fat in the diet, lying on the right side when resting or sleeping, and elevating the head of the bed may be enough to solve the problem. A new medication, metaclopromide, is now available and may give excellent relief. In addition, this is one situation in which just one injection of NPH insulin in the morning may be the best schedule since food is only gradually made available to the body.

Learning to live with diabetes rather than for it

Try hard not to let diabetes run your life or your family. It is not easy to keep your courage and patience, and you have a right to support and appreciation for the extra job you have to do every day. But your goal should be to be as efficient and cheerful as possible about your diabetes. When you become expert, you should not need more than half an hour a day for testing and injection, even if you are taking three or more injections a day. As life progresses, you will become skillful in how to find out whether a new problem is the result of the diabetes or is part of the nor-

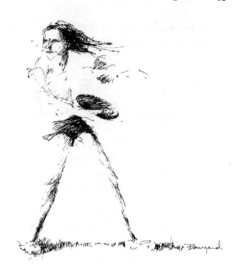

See how much better I feel on three or more injections a day.

mal ups and downs of an average life cycle. Review Chapter 7 for some suggestions and perspective.

Care of equipment and methods for insulin injection

Hundreds of thousands of people have been taking daily insulin injections since 1921. Over the years, it has been demonstrated that it is very important that both the skin and the equipment be very clean. However, they need not be "sterile." In fact, it is impossible to sterilize the skin. It is, however, essential to avoid contamination of the insulin bottle itself and of the interior of the syringe and needle. We have described the various options for drawing up and giving insulin with this in mind and with the desire to make your daily routines as practical, inexpensive, and flexible as possible.

Today, infections at the site of injection are very rare. They usually occur only if there is diabetes with long-standing neglect and resulting damage to the circulation and the skin tissues, or in cases of marked neglect of personal hygiene. These are the principles to keep in mind:

1. Infections are to be avoided because they can cause diabetes to become severe.
2. The insulin bottle is sterile and must remain so.

3. The needle must not touch anything because it goes into the insulin bottle and into your skin.
4. The inside of the barrel of the syringe and the plunger must also be kept "sterile" because they push air into the bottle and insulin into you.
5. You can't make your skin truly "sterile," but since the needle goes through it, it must be as clean as possible.

Insulin

Recently, it has been decided to have a new single strength of insulin, U100, and to develop special low-dose, narrow-gauge syringes for the people who only take a few units at a time. Therefore, U100 syringes have replaced U40 and U80 syringes.

Several companies make insulin and syringes. It is very important for you to know what insulin and syringes your doctor wants you to have. A description of the various types of insulin preparations and the length of time for which they are active is included in Chapter 11.

Your supply of insulin bottles should be stored in the refrigerator, where they will keep for more than a year. Do not use any insulin bottles after the "expiration date" stamped on the label. However, in an emergency you could probably safely use outdated insulin for several weeks or months beyond the expiration date.

The bottle you are using every day can be carried with you or left on a shelf in the house as long as it is not in the sun, next to a radiator or stove, or allowed to freeze.

Syringes

Syringes are available in glass or plastic. Detachable needles are available in steel or in plastic and steel with a plastic sheath or cover. Most people today use disposable plastic syringes. But they are more expensive.

To clean glass syringes and steel needles, take them apart and boil them for 5 minutes in a covered pan. The water can then be drained off and the syringe can remain in the covered pan until the time of your next injection. Then you can put the plunger back inside the syringe without touching the plunger. Attach the needle and lay it down on a safe clean surface so that the needle does not touch anything. One of the best ways to protect the needle is to use a plastic needle cover. Disposable needles can also be purchased to use with the glass syringe.

If you take more than one injection a day and need to carry equipment with you to school or work or when traveling, you may prefer to use disposable syringes. Since these are made of plastic, they should not be boiled because heat will cause them to warp.

Instructions on the package suggest that it is best to use a new disposable syringe for each injection. However, many people use disposable syringes more than once to cut cost and increase convenience. With very careful technique there is a very low risk of infection, especially if the person is basically active, healthy, and clean in personal habits.

Here are the important things to know

1. Never draw anything but sterile insulin back into the barrel.
2. Never touch the tip of the needle or let it hit anything.
3. Never remove the plunger or touch it.
4. After each use, immerse the needle in alcohol and put it back in its protective sheath while it is still wet with alcohol.
5. *Do not use disposable syringes more than once if you or anyone who lives or works with you has an infection.*

There are various brands of syringes to choose from, and they are continually being redesigned for convenience and quality. The short 27- and 28-gauge needles are very sharp and practically painless to use. Be sure to discuss the various brands with your nurse or physician and find the one you like best.

It is wise to have extra syringes and needles with you at home and when you travel in case of breakage or contamination. All your supplies will be less expensive if you buy them in quantity. If you qualify for Medicare or Medicaid, in many states the *cost of your supplies can be covered if you ask your physician to write a prescription for them.*

Insulin injection: timing and technique

The timing of your insulin injection in relation to your meals is an important factor in making it effective. This is where SBGM is a valuable ally. If possible, plan to test 40 to 60 minutes before your next meal. If your blood glucose level is over 200, take your insulin immediately. If your blood glucose level is near normal, between 70 and 150, wait for half an hour. Obviously, if your blood glucose level is on the low side, eat enough to prevent an insulin reaction and delay the injection until 5 to 10 minutes before the meal.

In general, take your insulin 20 to 30 minutes before a meal whenever possible.

1. If you are using long-acting cloudy insulins or a mixture of insulins, refer to the next section on mixing insulins.
2. Wipe off the cap of the insulin bottle with a cotton ball, pad, or clean facial tissue wetted with alcohol.
3. If you are using a plastic syringe, peel open the paper wrapper from the top and remove the plunger and needle cover. Save these items if you plan to reuse the syringe.
4. Pull the plunger back to the unit marking your dose. The syringe is now filled with air.
5. Invert the insulin bottle and push the needle into the rubber bottle cap.
6. Push the plunger so that the air is pushed inside the bottle.
7. Pull back the plunger to two or three units *above* your dosage mark, making sure that your insulin is going into the barrel of your syringe.
8. Remove any bubbles of air by flicking the syringe with your finger. Then push the plunger back to your dosage mark. It would not be harmful to inject air into your body, but you want to be sure that air does not change the dosage.
9. Take the needle out of the bottle gently, being sure that no insulin is lost.
10. Place the syringe on any surface, being sure that the needle does not touch anything.
11. If your skin is not clean, wipe it off with a spiral motion with the alcohol ball or soap and water, working from the center out. Insulin may be injected into the thighs, the buttocks, the abdomen, or the upper arms. It is a good idea to rotate the places where you inject insulin, using a different site each time, at least an inch apart. This provents local toughening of the skin and reduces the hollowing effect of frequent insulin injections. Today's insulins produce much less hollowing, if any.
12. To avoid putting the needle into muscle, pinch the skin up with one hand, using a wide grasp. If you are using your upper arm, you can lean against a door to push the skin up.
13. Adjust the syringe in your other hand so that the needle is pointed toward the skin. With the new short needle, the best angle is straight down. Push it in.
14. Many people pull back on the plunger to see if blood comes into

the barrel of the syringe. If blood appears, remove the syringe and change to another spot because the needle has punctured a blood vessel. The short needle usually only reaches the very smallest blood vessels, so it is not likely to be harmful. But if the insulin should go directly into a major blood vessel, a rapid severe insulin reaction could occur.

15. Press on the plunger to inject the insulin at an even rate into the tissue.
16. Remove the needle. Wipe the skin again if you want to do so.
17. Remember: Change the needle if anything at all has touched it before you have given yourself your insulin.
18. You can alternate using arms, legs, buttocks, and abdomen, taking into consideration the convenience of different sites according to whether you are at home or traveling. Of course, it is easier to use an arm instead of buttocks in a public place. Remember that insulin is absorbed fastest from the abdomen.

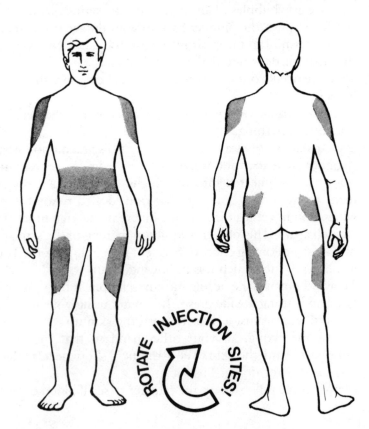

mixing insulins

If your physician has prescribed a mixture of insulins, be sure you know *how many units of each insulin* are to be taken and *how many units are in the total mixture*. Always mix insulins that are of the *same concentration*.

1. Prepare equipment as for a single dose. Place both vials of insulin before you.
2. Into the vial of cloudy insulin, inject an amount of air equal to the volume of the dose to be withdrawn from that vial. Pull the needle out of the stopper without withdrawing the insulin. This puts air pressure into the bottle for later.
3. Inject air into the vial of clear insulin, equal in volume to the dose to be withdrawn from this vial.
4. Turn the bottle of clear insulin upside down with the syringe still in it. Keep the end of the needle under the level of insulin in the bottle. This prevents drawing air into the syringe and cuts down on bubbles. Withdraw the specified dose.
5. Reinsert needle into the vial of cloudy insulin and withdraw whatever amount is required to make up the total dose of the mixture. Watch for air bubbles so that you do not push clear insulin into the cloudy insulin bottle.
6. Proceed with the injection.

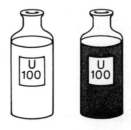

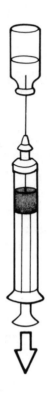

7. If a mixture of lente or semilente is prescribed, follow the same routine. The order of withdrawal makes no difference, *but be sure you know the proper dose of each insulin and the total amount of the mixed dose*. It is easiest to withdraw the insulins in the same order every time.

Traveling kit

Buy a small (5 x 6 inches) plastic-lined case, purse, or pouch to hold:
1. A very small bottle with alcohol and a few facial tissues or wipes
2. More than one syringe and some extra detachable needles
3. More than one bottle of insulin, in case of breakage
4. Diastix and Acetest tablets and blood testing equipment
5. Glucagon (especially if you are an unstable diabetic)

Chapter 14
PEEP in Type I diabetes

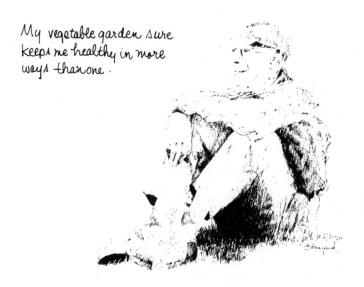

My vegetable garden sure keeps me healthy in more ways than one.

Physical activity for the insulin-dependent person

Exercise is one of your greatest allies for overall health and satisfaction. It will help you in achieving all your goals for a long and happy life. It will keep you in the running with your peers, bring you new friends and experiences, and teach you how to read your body signs so that you can adjust your daily routines to match your needs.

However, exercise for Type I diabetes does not have the important therapeutic role in self-care that it does for Type II diabetes where it can help to put the disorder into the background. An exercise program for insulin-dependent people aims to allow those who want to compete in sports or who enjoy physically active hobbies to exercise safely. People who take insulin should not exercise when their diabetes is out of control. But there is every reason to enjoy exercise when you are in reasonable control, provided you know how to plan for it. As we said in Chapter 3, to be physically active and strong is good for everyone for overall mental and bodily health. Here are some hints to keep in mind as you develop the exercise part of your PEEP.

Research has now shown without a doubt that a well-exercised person has body cells that respond quickly to small amounts of insulin. This is especially true for muscle and liver cells where the action of insulin is very important. Olympic athletes have very low levels of insulin in their blood even though they eat a great deal. Carbohydrates in food are burned easily by active muscles. You can see, therefore, that if you exercise regularly and vigorously two or three times a week, your overall insulin requirements will go down and your diet plan will be freer.

If you are a lean, active, essentially healthy insulin-dependent diabetic person, the chances are that your only handicap in regard to physical activity is anxiety over insulin reactions. There are two things to remember in this regard. First, it is the unusual person taking insulin who never has a reaction, even when everyone involved is trying to do the best they can with "control." So you are not alone, and you should not feel guilty if a reaction occurs. Second, insulin reactions can be prevented or minimized. They need not be anything more than a temporary inconvenience if they are properly handled. When a reaction does take place, it is encouraging to remember that the body's systems for raising blood glucose levels to normal are usually still functioning. Please refer to the section on insulin reactions for more detail.

Probably one of the greatest obstacles to good management of insulin-dependent diabetes is the concept that to take sugar in any form is to break your diet. If you have been led to believe this, replace that myth right now with the fact that energy output calls for food intake. You have insulin in your system like a nondiabetic person, and if you are exercising more than usual, you need more than the usual amount of quick energy calories, just like a nondiabetic person. The only difference lies in the fact that you need to keep closer track of the whole process, mentally.

There are two kinds of events for which the insulin-dependent diabetic needs to be prepared: planned sports events and unplanned demands on your energies. There is one easy way to avoid trouble in either case.

Carry concentrated sweets in some form with you wherever you go, even at home. Don't wait to learn this technique by having a close scrape with a bad accident at work, in sports, or while driving a car. These days, everyone eats at times on the run and between or instead of meals, so you won't even appear "different" in any way. Remember, too, that extra calories eaten in relation to exercise need not be counted in the diet.

It is surprising how much exercise may be involved in apparently routine activities such as shoveling the car out of a snowbank, mowing the lawn, or harvesting the family vegetable garden. If you are a young parent, you may bring on an insulin reaction running around caring for a family of sick children. *Be sure you take the time for your between-meal snacks.*

In addition to eating extra food, you can learn to reduce your insulin dose before planned, vigorous exercise such as a mountain hike, a long bike ride, or a tennis match. Insulin can be reduced anywhere from 20% to 80%, depending on you as an individual and the type of activity involved. Each individual has to experiment to find out how much, how often, and what combination of calories to eat and what to do about the dose of insulin. Of course, this is where SBGM can help, not only in making decisions at the beginning of the day, but in keeping track of blood glucose as the exercise continues. Keeping records as you experiment will teach you what to expect on a reflex basis.

A short period of vigorous exercise can bring down a moderately high blood sugar level without extra insulin. Jogging during coffee breaks is a great way to stay alert if you have an unusually long sedentary day. However, if you are in a *period of poor control with a blood sugar level over 300 and some ketones in the urine, exercise is not effective and extra insulin is necessary.*

In regard to competitive sports in general, people with insulin-dependent diabetes can teach themselves to engage in any sports to their liking. A few really exceptional people have become tennis champions, marathon runners, and members of professional football and baseball teams, such as Catfish Hunter. However, there are many other sports that may be more suitable for insulin-sensitive people or those in an older age group. Dancing is wonderful indoor exercise for winter. Many people enjoy cross-country skiing, swimming, hiking, and cycling. Just plain walking is very good exercise. Classes in yoga will make your body stronger and more flexible as well as bringing you tranquility.

Remember that your body can remain extra sensitive to insulin for 24 to 36 hours after an event. You may need to reduce your insulin the next day or so.

All the benefits of exercise can be yours. Go to it!

Nutrition for Type I people who are lean and active, young or adult

You have been told that your dietary needs don't differ from anyone else's and that the nutritional guidelines given to individuals with insulin-dependent diabetes are the same goals for everyone for optimal nutritional quality. Why then does eating become so frustrating at times?

If we look at what influences eating habits, we soon discover that food choices are not always determined by "what is good for us." There are many social, cultural, and psychological factors that are interrelated everytime we have a bite to eat. Reflect for a moment on what foods are associated with holidays in your home or meals that are considered the family favorites. Consider what foods are available for after-school snacks, getting together with friends, watching television, or having to eat when you're not hungry. All of these seemingly innocent situations do have more of an impact on you than on people who don't have diabetes. You have to think ahead. What was my blood sugar this morning? Am I going to exercise this afternoon or sit and read instead? Will I get home in time for dinner, or do I need to bring something along? That process limits freedom of choice and takes some of the fun out of daily life.

Allowing yourself to identify your feelings associated with eating may help you consider ways to cope with them. You need to develop your own specific guidelines around eating that we have referred to as PEEP. It will help you to make the right decisions about food with a minimum of frustration. In Chapter 2, we focused on what food is and how to look at food from a scientific point of view. In this chapter, we will look at possible ways to apply this information to your life-style.

The overall goals of a food plan for any insulin-dependent person are:

1. To develop a reasonably consistent pattern of eating throughout the day on which to base your schedule of insulin injections. This pattern will make it as easy and predictable as possible for you to think for your pancreas.
2. To eat sufficient food to grow normally and to maintain your level of activity.
3. To maintain an ideal body weight.
4. To avoid big swings of blood sugar to high (*hyper*glycemia) or low (*hypo*glycemia) levels.

The amount of food an insulin-dependent diabetic needs to reach these goals varies with age, stage of growth, level of physical activity, lifestyle, and general state of health. With the help of your diet counselor, you will work out your own food plan. There are several positive reasons for having a food plan or diet:

1. People with diabetes have to be smarter than most people about food. A diet plan can aid you in learning what you have to know about what is in various foods.

2. A food plan can help you to avoid sudden changes in the composition of your diet. You will find out how to balance meals so that there is the best combination of proteins, carbohydrates, and fats spaced evenly throughout the day.

3. You will learn how to think about food in relation to physical activity.

Please review Chapter 2.

Let's start out with a few words about the need for sugar in the diet. Before insulin was discovered, the only treatment for diabetes was to avoid sugar in all forms. We have the habit of thinking of sugar as dangerous or as a "poison." But we know that the primary fuel of the normal body is the form of sugar called glucose and that sugar in its simple or complex forms is essential for energy, much as gasoline is to an engine. It is very important for insulin-dependent diabetics to learn how and when to use and enjoy different forms of sugars in the diet. *The person who is taking insulin is really like a normal person in all requirements for food, except that the regulation of body fuels is not automatic.*

For the sake of developing good habits of eating, you and your diet counselor will decide on a food plan that sets a pattern and a limit for the overall amount of sugars and carbohydrates for everyday living. You will learn how to space the carbohydrates throughout the day so that you will have enough for your energy needs but not so much at any one time to cause the blood sugar to rise too high.

Then you will learn how to change your basic food plan to meet your needs when you are exercising, traveling, working overtime, or eating on an unusual schedule. For example, you need more carbohydrate when you are exercising and less when you are not. Changes can be made by eating between meals or by increasing or decreasing the amount taken at meals. Because it is not always possible to tell when extra food may be needed, it is important to know what snack foods are good for you and how to carry them with you at all times. There is more detail about this in other sections of this chapter (see "How to Live With Insulin Reactions," "Portable Snacks," and "Physical Activity").

In general, your diet should be balanced, that is, it should contain certain regular amounts of *protein* (meat, fish, eggs, cheese, dried beans, nuts, peanut butter, and milk), *fat* (margarine, oil, salad dressing, mayonnaise, bacon) and *carbohydrates* (fruits, vegetables, breads, cereals, rice, macaroni, noodles, potatoes). The amounts of each of these types of foods should be worked out for you *individually* with your diet counselor. Insofar as possible, try to eat your regular meals and any other *planned* between-meal or bedtime snacks at approximately the same time each day, much as you take your insulin at the same times each day. However, we all know that this is not always possible, so you must plan ahead as best you can to keep a reasonably regular schedule of eating. Learn how to compensate for weekend schedules of sleeping, eating, and activity that may be very different from the weekday school or work schedule. Remember that your eating schedule, and even your insulin schedule, can be changed to some degree to allow for these times. However, you may not be able to sleep in until noon without spoiling the way you feel for the rest of the day. In the beginning you will need the advice of your diet counselor or doctor, but with experience, you will learn to do it on your own.

Eating in a cafeteria at school or work can be a problem. Many cafeterias serve inexpensive food, which usually means it is high in sugars, starches, and fats and low in protein. However, if you know approximately what makes up a certain item on the menu, it is usually possible to make a "balanced" meal. After a little study, it is not very difficult to judge what a food item contains in terms of protein, carbohydrates, and fats. An example of this at a school lunch might be:

> Sloppy joe (protein, fat) on a
> Buttered bun (carbohydrate, fat) with
> Carrot sticks (carbohydrate)
> Ice cream (carbohydrate, fat, and protein)
> Milk (protein, carbohydrate, and fat if not skim)

You will soon know what quantity of each of the above items is the right amount to eat at a meal.

One of the best indications that tells your doctor or your diet counselor that you have your diabetes in good control is to know that you are keeping a *steady* weight for your height or are growing normally. If you lose weight it may mean you are not getting enough insulin or are having too little food, or both. That is a kind of starvation. However, if you are gaining weight out of proportion to your growth, it *always* means you are eating too much in relation to your physical activity. This *may* not be your fault, because if you are taking too much insulin, you may just be protecting yourself from insulin reactions by overeating. Insulin helps to make body fat out of excess food of *any* type that you eat. So total calories and amount of any foods *are* important. This is a matter for you and your doctor to talk over.

Remember what we said at the beginning of this section: The person with diabetes who is taking insulin is really like a normal person in all requirements for food, except that the regulation of body fuels is not automatic. *You have to do the thinking for the pancreas.*

How to live with insulin reactions

Low blood glucose, hypoglycemia, often called insulin reaction, is described in Tables 7 through 9 in terms of what may cause it and how it feels in comparison with high blood glucose. Of course, it is important to avoid both extremes as much as possible, not only because they are unpleasant and tiring but also because they are unhealthy. However, when someone takes enough insulin to control the diabetes, it may be almost impossible to avoid occasional insulin reactions. Therefore, it is helpful to know how to handle them. In fact, some physicians prefer that people recently diagnosed as having diabetes have an insulin reaction right away, to learn what their own symptoms are, for practice and experience. Insulin reactions happen even when both the diabetic person and the health team are doing their best to control the blood glucose. At this stage in knowledge, we all have to accept this, and two good things happen when we do so: (1) no one is accused of cheating, and people learn to cope without fear or guilt; and (2) the doctor or nurse is not blamed unfairly for not providing the best treatment.

In order not to be anxious, it is comforting to know that, for the average, healthy, active diabetic, an insulin reaction does not lead to coma and death. Low blood glucose levels may lead to loss of judgment and even temporary unconsciousness, which could be dangerous if untreated. However, all the body's automatic systems for restoring the blood to normal are still functioning although they may be blunted. In most instances, recovery is complete within a short time even if unconsciousness occurs.

The best hope of *preventing reactions during planned exercise* is to eat enough of the right kind of extra calories beforehand, throughout, and after the period to give you that short- and long-term energy you need. (Please review the section on physical activity at the beginning of this chapter.) To provide carbohydrates, protein, and fat, many athletes eat a peanut butter and jelly sandwich with milk before exercise. During exercise, some people need to eat fruit or candy every half hour, especially during a lively tennis game or mountain hike. Many people also need extra food or less insulin the day after an athletic event.

It is particularly important to be on the *alert to periods of unplanned activity,* such as washing storm windows or cars, hanging out laundry on a windy day, or moving furniture. Keep some food handy in your pockets and think ahead as much as possible each day.

Of course, if you are planning to exercise to bring down a high blood sugar level, you do not need to eat anything extra!

The way to *recover from or stop an insulin reaction* is to learn how it feels and immediately to eat enough concentrated sweets to raise your blood glucose level. In practice, this means having at hand sugar in any form that you prefer, wherever you go. The kind of sweets you use may vary according to your taste, where you live and work, and also the season of the year. For example, chocolate is messy in hot weather and orange juice is sloppy if you are changing storm windows on a ladder! See the section on portable snacks for suggestions.

Insulin reactions vary in symptoms and length, not only from one person to another, but from time to time for each individual. There is no rule of thumb as to how much you should eat. Usually, especially as you become skilled at picking up the first sensations, a few ounces of juice, perhaps with a tablespoon of sugar, may be enough. On rare occasions, you may need 2 to 3 times that much and still feel hungry when you are over the worst of it. Your appetite is a good guide in most cases, and you will not do yourself any harm if you eat somewhat more than the juice and sugar usually recommended. In fact, it is a good idea to eat some protein along with the sugar for longer protection, especially if you plan to continue doing whatever you were doing after you have recovered. You do not need to include in your diet plan the calories you ate to correct a low blood glucose level, so exercise does allow you to liberalize your diet. But, of course, binges of eating extra calories are always to be avoided.

Quite frequently there is a period after a reaction when the control of your diabetes is temporarily poor. Urine tests may show some sugar. This is not usually a result of what you ate during the reaction, but the result of the body's normal sugar-producing responses. It is important *not* to increase your insulin to make up for this temporary high blood sugar level, because you may then have another reaction.

Sometimes people have prolonged reactions without knowing it, especially at night when asleep. These reactions may also produce temporary high urine and blood glucose levels, again because of the body's sugar-producing response to the reaction. If you are restless at night and wake in the morning with a headache and a high urine sugar level, that may mean that you are having unnoticed insulin reactions. Check with your physician. (See Chapter 13.)

Once we understand the system, we do not need to be afraid. You, an insulin-dependent diabetic, *can carry your pancreas with you in your pocket instead of in the body*. With sugar, insulin, and exercise at hand at all times, most people with diabetes can be essentially normal, fully active, and not at risk of anything more than temporary discomfort.

Table 7 provides warning signs, Table 8 provides causes and symptoms, and Table 9 provides treatment and prevention measures for both types of insulin reaction.

Remember to check your sugar supplies every day!!!

Table 7. How can you tell which reaction is taking place?

Warning signs	Low blood sugar: insulin reaction	High blood sugar: diabetic acidosis
Skin	Pale, moist	Flushed, dry
Behavior	Excited, nervous, irritable, confused	Drowsy
Breath	Normal	Fruity odor
Breathing	Normal to rapid, shallow	Deep, labored
Vomiting	Absent	Present
Tongue	Moist, numb, tingling	Dry
Hunger	Present	Absent
Thirst	Absent	Present
Pain	Headache	Abdominal
Sugar in urine	Absent or slight	Large amounts
Vision	Blurry, double	Normal

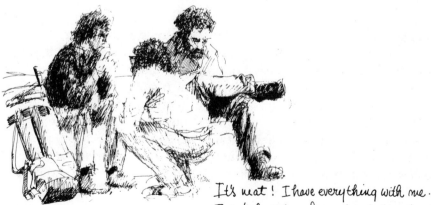

*It's neat! I have everything with me.
I don't have to go home for food or insulin!*

Table 8. How can you tell which reaction is taking place?

	Low blood sugar: insulin reaction	High blood sugar: diabetic acidosis
Causes	Too much insulin Too little food Excessive exercise without extra food	Too little insulin Omission of insulin Too much food Infection or fever Stress Surgery Neglect Not knowing what to do when problems occur Failure to treat positive urine or blood tests
Onset	Regular insulin—sudden, 2–3 hours after dose NPH, lente—slower, 6–8 hours after dose	Slow, gradual—hours, days
Warning symptoms	Dizziness Shakiness Tired Hungry Irritable Sweaty Pale Poor coordination Slurred speech Double vision Headache If untreated: stupor, convulsions	Nausea, vomiting Excessive thirst Headache Abdominal pain Excessive urination Dry skin Flushed Sweet, fruity breath Fatigue Deep, difficult breathing Confusion Coma

Glucagon

Glucagon is the hormone produced by alpha cells in the pancreas. It raises blood sugar levels by breaking down glycogen stored in the liver and also by speeding the conversion of protein to glucose in the liver. It is now available for injection much like insulin. It comes in two bottles, one with dried glucagon, and the other with sterile fluid to dissolve it. It can be very useful to have with you in case you have a very severe reaction, especially if you are traveling or camping. Ask your doctor to prescribe it for you. Be sure that someone teaches a *friend or member of your family how to use it* in case you are unconscious, just as someone should

Table 9. Treatment and prevention

	Low blood sugar: insulin reaction	High blood sugar: diabetic acidosis

Treatment	Fast-acting sugars
	   Sugar cubes, 2
	   Orange juice, ½ cup
	   Sweet soft drink, ½ cup
	   Honey, Karo, 2 teaspoons
	   Glutose or Instant Glucose
	Glucagon injection in emergency
	Intravenous glucose in ambulance
	   or hospital
		Test urine frequently for sugar
		   and ketones
		Contact physician; may need
		   adjustment in insulin dose
		Severe acidosis requires
		   hospitalization

Prevention	1. Don't skip meals 2. Avoid sudden changes in insulin, exercise, and food 3. Before extra exercise, take slow-acting carbohydrate 4. Always carry some form of sugar with you to treat early signs 5. Discuss change of insulin dose with your physician if reactions are frequent 6. Educate family and friends in what to look for and how to treat 7. Wear identification 8. Have regular check-ups	1. Always take *some* insulin 2. Test urine regularly and keep record 3. When showing ketones, increase fluid intake and test urine more often 4. Contact physician if ketones are strongly positive or increasing 2 or 3 times in a row 5. Wear identification 6. Have regular check-ups

know how to give you insulin in an emergency. If you are unable to swallow because of unconsciousness, Glutose or cake frosting can be squeezed between the cheek and gum, where it will dissolve and be absorbed.

Portable snacks and quick meals for the insulin-dependent person

Life for the insulin-dependent person can be almost as flexible as anyone else's—if food and insulin are always available. Today, there are many foods that are easy to carry, and because of the way everyone moves around today, the diabetic who is eating on the run is not any different from others.

Healthy, nutritious snacks are available at many counters in packaged forms such as sesame bars and small boxes of raisins or cheese crackers.

However, you can make up your own both for variety and to lower the cost. In addition, campers' supply stores and natural food stores have many interesting and nourishing dried foods that are suitable.

You should really carry food of two types. One is to substitute for a delayed meal and should have protein, fat, and carbohydrate. The other is concentrated sweets to prevent or recover from an insulin reaction.

> *Snacks containing protein, fat, and carbohydrate*
> Cheese and peanut butter with crackers
> Dried fruits and nuts, mixed
> Dried beef
> Campers' hard chocolate
> Sesame bars, granola bars, Pillsbury Foodsticks
> Gorp: mixture of cold cereals with dried fruits, nuts, crackers
> *Snacks as concentrated sweets*
> Dried fruit or fruit rolls
> Small cans of fruit juice
> Hard candy, individually wrapped, or gum drops, Necco wafers, Lifesavers
> Envelopes or lumps of sugar to dissolve in water or juice
> Molasses and peanut butter kisses
> Tube of cake frosting
> Commercial jellies such as Glutose

In addition to portable snacks, a handy collection of quick, easy-to-prepare meals can be helpful. You may want to have a couple of recipes in which all the ingredients can be stored on hand either in the cupboard or the freezer for those unexpected days when you are delayed in coming home. When you use these ingredients, be sure to replace them! If you know what your plans are at the beginning of the day, you can use a crockpot to prepare a meal while you are away from home. Microwave ovens also help to make food available in a hurry.

The evening meal is not the only challenge. Breakfast often gets squeezed in while running out the door for work or school. This is a very important meal both in terms of managing your diabetes and in starting the body out properly for energy that will last through the day. Some suggestions for breakfast on the run are yogurt with fruit and cereal (bran buds offer a little crunchy taste), bran muffin with peanut butter, or pocket bread and cheese. Use your imagination to think of new combinations for each meal of the day. There are many cookbooks that are geared to "meals in minutes." Ask your local library or affiliate and your diet counselor for help.

Chapter 15
Health maintenance and sick day guidelines

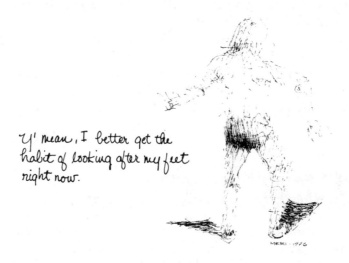

Y' mean, I better get the habit of looking after my feet right now.

MERI·1976

General sick day guidelines

Your diabetes will change as your body responds to the stress of illness. Because illness may affect you in different ways, depending on the part of the body most severely involved, there are no rules that fit every situation. For this reason, it is important for you *to get in touch with your doctor or nurse whenever you are out of control* because of illness to establish the routines for the sickness. It is really easier for everyone if you do this right away. Of course, some minor ailments, such as a mild cold, bring about little or no change in your diabetes. But others, such as a bacterial infection that causes boils or a severe intestinal virus, can rapidly make the diabetes worse.

Two important principles

1. Check every urine specimen for both glucose and ketones. Call your doctor if you have moderate or strong indication of acetone. Check your blood every 2 hours.

2. Be sure to take enough insulin to meet your minimal needs, especially until you reach your doctor for further advice. *You still need insulin even if you are not eating.* Your body will continue to feed itself by breaking down its stored energy. Therefore, insulin is as essential as ever to utilize the glucose and fat stores being released into your bloodstream. Remember how you felt when your diabetes was first diagnosed, before you got your insulin? You won't want to add that feeling to the misery of your present illness! *Check supplies on hand* at regular intervals:

   a. Some regular insulin, in case you need to be on several injections a day for a while

   b. Sweet juices and sodas such as ginger ale, cola, apple juice, Kool-aid; clear broth; tea; saltines

   c. Glucagon, the injectable hormone that raises the blood sugar level (see Chapter 14)

Specific directions if your illness affects your ability to eat

The important thing is to have just enough insulin to avoid acidosis. Since your body is changing all the time, it is necessary to watch all the signs by taking frequent tests and to be able to correct quickly to avoid an insulin reaction. The easiest way to do this may be to take insulin more often and in smaller doses than usual, under the direction of your doctor.

If you wake in the morning nauseated and barely able to eat and are unable to reach your doctor:

1. Take half of your usual morning dose of insulin all in the form of *regular* or *semi-lente* insulin. If your urine test is moderately or strongly positive for acetone, take a maximum of 25 units, or two thirds of your usual morning dose. If you inject the insulin into the muscle in the upper arm, it will be absorbed more rapidly.

2. Take a light feeding of one of the following, according to your tolerance:

   a. A light hot cereal with sugar

   b. Skim milk with sugar added (1 tablespoon to each glass)

    c. Sweetened drinks such as ginger ale, cola, Kool-aid, or tea

    d. Plain ginger ale

3. Check each voided urine for both glucose and acetone. Keep a running record, including an estimate of the amount voided.

4. *If you are unable to eat at all, call your physician without delay.* If he or she is unavailable, go to a clinic or hospital emergency room. You need glucose along with insulin to keep you out of ketosis. *If you are unable to take anything by mouth, you must obtain assistance.*

5. If you are actively vomiting, do *not* continue to drink liquids, since this will withdraw salts from your body.

6. If you have diarrhea, take broth (beef or chicken), saltines, and orange juice to replace the lost sodium and potassium.

If there is unavoidable delay in reaching medical aid, you can stay out of serious trouble if:

1. You take small doses of *regular insulin,* 10 to 20 units every 4 hours while checking your urine and blood.

2. If you are clear of glucose and acetone, take sugar-containing fluids, as above, and less than 10 units of insulin.

3. If vomiting persists, try taking a tablespoon of Kool-aid made with sugar every 5 minutes.

4. If urine tests show acetone *plus* a large volume of urine with over 2% glucose, you have become temporarily insulin-resistant. You may need 25 or more units of regular insulin at a time.

Once you have learned these skills, you and your doctor can "talk you through an illness on the telephone" and you can avoid going to the hospital.

Foot care for young people

Care of the foot is important for everyone, so these recommendations apply not only to people with diabetes. Good habits save trouble later!

Your feet are strong and well-formed, and you want to keep them that way. Look at your feet every day in the same way that you comb your hair and brush your teeth.

Everyday care

1. It is hard to keep the feet clean, but it is necessary because healing takes longer than in other parts of the body. Infection can start more easily in moist, dirty feet. Wash your feet often. Clean, cotton socks keep moisture at a minimum.

2. Be sure that your shoes and socks fit well, allowing for growth.
3. Wear shoes that are suitable for whatever activity is planned. When you are barefoot, choose the terrain very carefully.
4. Be sure your tetanus shot is up to date. You need a booster every 10 years or after injury if you have not had one within 1 year.
5. Watch out for rashes, warts, athlete's foot, calluses, and splinters.
6. Cut your nails carefully, straight across the top and not too short.
7. If you have had diabetes for more than 10 years, you should take particular care of your feet. Follow the instructions concerning foot care in Chapter 10.

Sports

1. If you are a winter sports fan, be sure to protect your feet from the cold. Avoid tight boots and wear several layers of absorbent socks (cotton or wool).
2. Be sure to buy comfortably fitting shoes and boots and break in new foot gear slowly enough to avoid blisters. This is especially true for hiking and ski boots. Use moleskin to protect vulnerable spots and prevent blisters.
3. In case of injury, first aid measures should be used immediately. Infection is easier to prevent and to treat than before the days of antibiotics, but infections make your diabetes more difficult to manage.
4. If your feet are injured when you are away from home, be sure to tell people that you have diabetes.
5. It is a good idea to carry some Band-Aids and antiseptic ointment with you as part of your travel kit of insulin, syringes, testing materials, and extra food.
6. Tell your doctor if there is anything unusual or painful about your feet.

Wear your identification emblem at all times!

Pregnancy in insulin-dependent diabetes

Pregnancy presents a real challenge to the management of insulin-dependent diabetes. This challenge can be met today with the resources of maternal-fetal high-risk centers throughout the country and a high level of dedication in the mother-to-be. The challenge begins before conception. We now know enough about how the mother's nutrition nourishes the baby to recognize that wide swings in the blood sugar level and a rise in ketones in the blood will increase the chances of congenital defects in the baby. Since it is difficult to predict the exact time of conception, it is important to plan a period of very careful management of diabetes for a couple of months ahead of time.

The most important period of pregnancy from the point of view of the development of the baby is the first 3 months. It may not be easy to keep the blood glucose within normal ranges during the morning sickness phase of pregnancy, but it can be done with SBGM and multiple injections or the use of an insulin pump. These measures will have to be continued throughout pregnancy to balance the mother's and the baby's nutrition.

During the latter months of pregnancy, the mother's body makes nutrients available to the baby, often at the expense of the mother. Her tissues become resistant to insulin, and her ketones may rise in the blood as her body turns to fat for energy. When the mother's blood glucose level rises, it crosses the placenta to the baby and stimulates release of insulin from the baby. The combination of a high blood glucose level and increased insulin may produce abnormally large and fat infants.

Physical exercise is beneficial to people with insulin-dependent diabetes (see Chapter 14), and moderate exercise can be good preparation for pregnancy and be useful during pregnancy. However, an abrupt increase in the level of activity during pregnancy for a person who is not in good condition to begin with may affect the supply of blood to the uterus. Again, the message is, be in good condition before the pregnancy begins.

It is extremely important to be in touch with specialists in pregnancy and diabetes if you decide to become pregnant.

Chapter 16
Consumer skills for a lifelong challenge in a competitive world

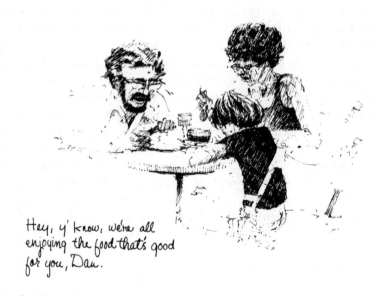

Hey, y' know, we're all enjoying the food that's good for you, Dan.

What to look for in a doctor

1. You have a right to choose and interview your doctor, and there are many from which to choose. The doctor does not have to be a diabetes specialist if he or she is interested in and up-to-date on diabetes.
2. Your doctor should be someone you like because it will be a long-term relationship.

3. Look for someone who likes to listen and who can share responsibilities for your treatment with you.
4. Be sure your doctor is interested in you as a whole human being, not just in blood tests. Your treatment should be unique to you as an individual.
5. Ask if your family can be included in instruction and in developing your plan for self-care and education.
6. Be sure your doctor knows who to refer you to for special needs such as eye exams, pregnancy, foot care, and community resources. Ask him or her to be the coordinator of your care.
7. Keep an eye out for physicians who have interactive video programs for self-education in their waiting rooms. Then you can test yourself, improve your skills, and share the results with your doctor. One such program now available is called Primarius, Inc., and is manufactured in San Diego.

The team approach

When you live with a lifelong problem like diabetes, you will need more advice and help than a physician alone can offer you. Many physicians and clinics recognize this and have developed what is called the team approach to care. A nurse and a diet counselor are usually on the team, and they, in turn, can reach people with other professional skills, such as ophthalmologists, obstetricians, podiatrists, social workers, and physical therapists. When this approach is really working well, the team members stay in touch about what they do for each individual. Care is coordinated, and the person who has diabetes takes part in all the decisions. If you live in an area where a formal team approach is not available, you can get much the same results yourself if you learn what to look for and what to ask for.

Join the American Diabetes Association!

How to judge what to believe and what to buy

Now that diabetes is recognized as a serious national health problem, a lot of money is being invested to capture the consumer market. There has been a great increase in the number of special foods and equipment that are supposed to simplify self-care. One of the most interesting skills you'll need is how to judge the quality of these items. The basic needs of anyone who has diabetes are expensive enough as it is. It is important to avoid buying unnecessary gadgets or misleading information. Here are some simple guidelines to help you to decide how to invest your money.

1. In regard to equipment, if you have basic questions about whether the item is necessary or reliable, call your local American Diabetes Association affiliate or the national office. Of course, when it comes to an instrument such as an insulin pump, your physician will be able to tell you which ones have been properly tested in a research situation on human beings.

2. In regard to books, articles, and films, be wary if the authors sound 100% certain that their programs are the complete answer. Look to see who sponsored the film or book. Check to see if there are references given to other people's work. There are no simple answers to complex questions. Far too little is known about how the human body adapts to use the energy in food. No one has the complete answers yet! Again, your local ADA is a good resource.

3. Shop around for the best prices. Consider group buying of basic items. Look for companies that offer bulk mailings direct to your home with automatic charging to your health insurance. Read the fine print!

Community resources

The person who lives with diabetes can make good use of many resources in most communities. Hospitals should offer ongoing diabetes education classes. Health spas, YMCAs, and YWCAs offer exercise programs. Dance, relaxation, yoga, and weight loss classes may be available. Your American Diabetes Association affiliate may have peer support groups, and if they don't, you can consider trying to get one started with guidance from their Patient Education Committee. Your pharmacist should be able to tell you a great deal about the self-care materials and medications now available. Use your imagination and the telephone book to enhance your care. Remember to share your plans with your physician, because you both need to have a complete, overall picture of your self-care.

Appendixes

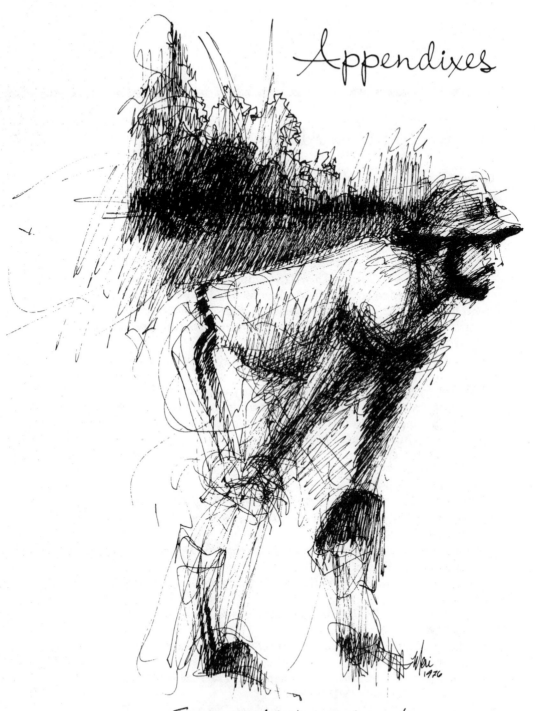

I've got a lot of experience to
offer. How can I help?

Appendix A

![section divider]

SUGGESTED READINGS

General

American Diabetes Association: *Diabetes '84,* a newsletter for those who live with diabetes'' (2 Park Ave., New York, NY 10016, free).

American Diabetes Association: *Diabetes Care* (for professionals and others interested in the practical application of research).

American Diabetes Association: *Diabetes in the Family,* Englewood Cliffs, N.J., 1982, Prentice-Hall, Inc. (The ADA comprehensive reference book on diabetes, addressed to both the newly diagnosed and those who have had diabetes for some time, and to their families. A valuable handbook of information on all aspects of diabetes, diagnosis, treatment, control, psychosocial impact, and the future of research.)

American Diabetes Association: *Diabetes Forecast* (your first and foremost reference, the magazine that has articles on every topic of interest from careers to cookery, insulins to insurance, pregnancy to parenting and peer support groups). Provided as a benefit of membership in ADA. To join ADA or to obtain a complete list of ADA materials, contact your local ADA affiliate or write to the national headquarters.

American Diabetes Association: *Guide to Good Living,* a pamphlet from the editors of *Diabetes Forecast.* (An A to Z guide for integrating good diabetes management into the life-style of the 1980s.)

American Diabetes Association: *The Kids' Corner,* New York, 1983.

Bierman, June, and Toohey, Barbara: *The Diabetic's Total Health Book,* Los Angeles, 1980, J.P. Tarcher, Inc.

Bierman, June, and Toohey, Barbara: *The Peripatetic Diabetic,* Boston, 1984, Houghton-Mifflin Co.

Colen, B.D.: *The Diabetic's 365-Day Medical Diary,* St. Louis, 1983, The C.V. Mosby Co.

Cousins, Norman: *The Healing Heart: Antidotes to Panic and Helplessness,* New York, 1983, W.W. Norton & Co., Inc.

Krall, Leo P., editor: *Joslin Diabetes Manual,* ed. 11, Philadelphia, 1978, Lea & Febiger.

National Diabetes Information Clearinghouse: *The Diabetes Dictionary,* 1983, Box NDIC, Bethesda, MD 20205.

Lodewick, Peter A.: *A Diabetic Doctor Looks at Diabetes: His and Yours,* Cambridge, Mass., 1982, RMI Corporation.

Fitness Through Physical Activity

Bierman, June, and Toohey, Barbara: *Cross-Country Skiing for the Fun of It,* New York, 1973, Dodd, Mead & Co.

Bierman, June, and Toohey, Barbara: *Diabetic's Sports and Exercise Book,* Philadelphia, 1977, J.P. Lippincott Co.

Cooper, Kenneth: *The New Aerobics,* New York, 1980, Bantam Books, Inc. (paperback).

Cookbooks and Meal Planning

American Diabetes Association and American Dietetic Association: *The Exchange Lists for Meal Planning,* New York, 1976.

American Diabetes Association and American Dietetic Association: *The Family Cookbook and Nutrition Guide,* vol. 1, 1980 and vol. 2, 1984, New York, Prentice-Hall, Inc.

American Diabetes Association and American Dietetic Association: *A Guide for Professionals: The Effective Application of Exchange Lists,* New York, 1977, The Associations.

American Diabetes Association and Metropolitan Center of Minneapolis: *Diabetes: Recipes for Health,* Maryland, 1983, Robert J. Brady Co.

Anderson, James W.: *The User's Guide to HCF Diet in Diabetes,* UK Diabetes Fund, 1872 Blairmoor Rd., Lexington, KY 40502.

Anderson, James W.: *Plant Fiber and Foods,* UK Diabetes Fund (Nutrient composition tables with information on calories, protein, fat, and dietary fiber).

Franz, Marion: *Fast Food Facts: Nutritive Values for Fast Food Restaurants,* 1983, International Diabetes Foundation, 4959 Education Blvd., Minneapolis, MN 55436 (Cost $2.50 plus shipping).

Inheritance and Pregnancy

American Diabetes Association: Giving Birth, *Diabetes Forecast,* reprint no. 323.

Type I Diabetes

Kleiman, Gary, and Doby, Sanford: *No Time To Lose,* New York, 1983, William Morrow & Co., Inc. (A personal story, dramatically told for young adult reading.)

Peterson, Charles M.: *Take Charge of Your Diabetes,* New York, 1979, Rockefeller University Press.

Pray, Lawrence: *Journey of a Diabetic,* New York, 1983, Simon & Schuster, Inc.

Travis, Luther B.: *An Instructional Aid to Juvenile Diabetes,* Galveston, Tex., 1982, University of Texas Medical Branch.

Type II Diabetes

Bailey, Covert: *Fit or Fat,* Boston, 1978, Houghton-Mifflin Co.

Jordan, Henry A., Levitz, Leonard S., and Kimbrell, Gordon M.: *Eating is OKAY! A Radical Approach to Successful Weight Loss,* Woburn, Mass., 1976, Butterworth Publishers, Inc.

Mahoney, M.J., and Mahoney, K.: *Permanent Weight Control,* New York, 1976, W.W. Norton & Co., Inc.

Sims, D.F., and Sims, E.A.H.: *The Other Diabetes,* New York, 1982, American Diabetes Association.

Stuart, R.B.: *Act Thin, Stay Thin,* New York, 1978, W.W. Norton & Co., Inc.

Appendix B

LOCATING THE AMERICAN DIABETES ASSOCIATION

NATIONAL OFFICE

American Diabetes Association
2 Park Avenue
New York, NY 10016
(212) 683-7444

Affiliate Associations of the American Diabetes Association (look in the white pages of your telephone book for addresses and phone numbers)

American Diabetes Association
Alabama Affiliate, Inc.
Huntsville, Alabama

American Diabetes Association
Alaska Affiliate, Inc.
Anchorage, Alaska

American Diabetes Association
Arizona Affiliate, Inc.
Phoenix, Arizona

American Diabetes Association
Arkansas Affiliate, Inc.
Little Rock, Arkansas

American Diabetes Association
Southern California Affiliate, Inc.
Los Angeles, California

American Diabetes Association
Northern California Affiliate, Inc.
San Francisco, California

American Diabetes Association
Colorado Affiliate, Inc.
Denver, Colorado

American Diabetes Association
Connecticut Affiliate, Inc.
West Hartford, Connecticut

American Diabetes Association
Delaware Affiliate, Inc.
Wilmington, Delaware

American Diabetes Association
Florida Affiliate, Inc.
Orlando, Florida

American Diabetes Association
Georgia Affiliate, Inc.
Atlanta, Georgia

American Diabetes Association
Hawaii Affiliate, Inc.
Honolulu, Hawaii

American Diabetes Association
Idaho Affiliate, Inc.
Boise, Idaho

American Diabetes Association
Maine Affiliate, Inc.
Augusta, Maine

American Diabetes Association
New Mexico Affiliate, Inc.
Albuquerque, New Mexico

American Diabetes Association
New York Diabetes Affiliate, Inc.
New York, New York

American Diabetes Association
New York State Affiliate, Inc.
Syracuse, New York

American Diabetes Association
North Carolina Affiliate, Inc.
Rocky Mount, North Carolina

American Diabetes Association
North Dakota Affiliate, Inc.
Grand Forks, North Dakota

American Diabetes Association
Akron Area Affiliate, Inc.
Akron, Ohio

American Diabetes Association
Cincinnati Affiliate, Inc.
Cincinnati, Ohio

American Diabetes Association
Dayton Area Affiliate, Inc.
Dayton, Ohio

American Diabetes Association
Greater Ohio Affiliate, Inc.
Perrysburgh, Ohio

American Diabetes Association
Oklahoma Affiliate, Inc.
Tulsa, Oklahoma

American Diabetes Association
Oregon Affiliate, Inc.
Portland, Oregon

American Diabetes Association
Mid-Pennsylvania Affiliate, Inc.
Bethlehem, Pennsylvania

American Diabetes Association
Greater Philadelphia Affiliate, Inc.
Philadelphia, Pennsylvania

American Diabetes Association
Western Penna. Affiliate, Inc.
Pittsburgh, Pennsylvania

American Diabetes Association
Northern Illinois Affiliate, Inc.
Chicago, Illinois

American Diabetes Association
Downstate Illinois Affiliate, Inc.
Decatur, Illinois

American Diabetes Association
Indiana Affiliate, Inc.
Indianapolis, Indiana

American Diabetes Association
Iowa Affiliate, Inc.
Cedar Rapids, Iowa

American Diabetes Association
Kansas Affiliate, Inc.
Wichita, Kansas

American Diabetes Association
Kentucky Affiliate, Inc.
Lexington, Kentucky

American Diabetes Association
Louisiana Affiliate, Inc.
Baton Rouge, Louisiana

American Diabetes Association
Maryland Affiliate, Inc.
Baltimore, Maryland

American Diabetes Association
Washington, D.C. Area Affiliate, Inc.
Silver Spring, Maryland

American Diabetes Association
Massachusetts Affiliate, Inc.
Newton Upper Falls, Massachusetts

American Diabetes Association
Michigan Affiliate, Inc.
Detroit, Michigan

American Diabetes Association
Minnesota Affiliate, Inc.
Minneapolis, Minnesota

American Diabetes Association
Mississippi Affiliate, Inc.
Jackson, Mississippi

American Diabetes Association
Missouri Regional Affiliate, Inc.
Columbia, Missouri

American Diabetes Association
Heart of America Affiliate, Inc.
Kansas City, Missouri

American Diabetes Association
Greater St. Louis Affiliate, Inc.
St. Louis, Missouri

American Diabetes Association
Montana Affiliate, Inc.
Great Falls, Montana

American Diabetes Association
Nebraska Affiliate, Inc.
Omaha, Nebraska

American Diabetes Association
Nevada Affiliate, Inc.
Las Vegas, Nevada

American Diabetes Association
New Hampshire Affiliate, Inc.
Concord, New Hampshire

American Diabetes Association
New Jersey Affiliate, Inc.
Bridgewater, New Jersey

American Diabetes Association
Rhode Island Affiliate, Inc.
Providence, Rhode Island

American Diabetes Association
South Carolina Affiliate, Inc.
Columbia, South Carolina

American Diabetes Association
South Dakota Affiliate, Inc.
Sioux Falls, South Dakota

American Diabetes Association
Memphis Mid-South Affiliate, Inc.
Memphis, Tennessee

American Diabetes Association
Greater Tennessee Affiliate, Inc.
Nashville, Tennessee

American Diabetes Association
Texas Affiliate, Inc.
Austin, Texas

American Diabetes Association
Utah Affiliate, Inc.
Salt Lake City, Utah

American Diabetes Association
Vermont Affiliate, Inc.
Burlington, Vermont

American Diabetes Association
Virginia Affiliate, Inc.
Charlottesville, Virginia

American Diabetes Association
Washington Affiliate, Inc.
Seattle, Washington

American Diabetes Association
West Virginia Affiliate, Inc.
Charleston, West Virginia

American Diabetes Association
Wisconsin Affiliate, Inc.
Milwaukee, Wisconsin

American Diabetes Association
Wyoming Affiliate, Inc.
Cheyenne, Wyoming

Membership in the American Diabetes Association is open to everyone. Over 200,000 people have participated in ADA efforts to fight diabetes. Benefits include a subscription to *Diabetes Forecast,* a diabetes newsletter containing information on local events and educational programs, and membership in the ADA affiliate nearest the member. To join, contact the American Diabetes Association, Membership Department, 2 Park Avenue, New York, NY 10016.

INDEX